METHODS IN MOLECULAR BIOLOGY

Series Editor
John M. Walker
School of Life and Medical Sciences
University of Hertfordshire
Hatfield, Hertfordshire, AL10 9AB, UK

For further volumes:
http://www.springer.com/series/7651

Extracellular RNA

Methods and Protocols

Edited by

Tushar Patel

Department of Transplantation, Mayo Clinic, Jacksonville, FL, USA

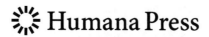 Humana Press

Editor
Tushar Patel
Department of Transplantation
Mayo Clinic
Jacksonville, FL, USA

ISSN 1064-3745   ISSN 1940-6029   (electronic)
Methods in Molecular Biology
ISBN 978-1-4939-8535-7   ISBN 978-1-4939-7652-2   (eBook)
https://doi.org/10.1007/978-1-4939-7652-2

Printed on acid-free paper

This Humana Press imprint is published by Springer Nature
The registered company is Springer Science+Business Media, LLC
The registered company address is: 233 Spring Street, New York, NY 10013, U.S.A.

Preface

Extracellular RNAs (exRNAs), RNA molecules found outside the cellular environment, are rapidly garnering attention as signaling mediators involved in intercellular communication and also for their potential as disease biomarkers or therapeutics. Cell-to-cell communication is a central component of cellular and tissue homeostasis, and development. Perturbation of these processes can contribute to the pathogenesis or progression of disease. RNA molecules can be released from cells but avoid degradation by incorporation within membrane bound vesicles (extracellular vesicles) or by association with lipids or proteins. Retention of their structural integrity contributes to retention of their biological effects. There are several different types of exRNA, with specificity based on their cells of origin and evidence of selective release into extracellular vesicles. They are found in the circulation and also in several biological fluids. Recognition of their diverse functional involvement in cellular processes and participation in cell and tissue development have all contributed to a rapidly growing interest in the field of exRNA.

The study of exRNA has been facilitated by the development of methods for the isolation and analysis of exRNA. Many of the methods and protocols in this book have been developed by groups supported by the Office of the NIH Director supported Common Fund program on Extracellular RNA. The resources and initiatives supported by this program have truly been a catalyst and galvanized research in exRNA.

The book is divided into four main sections, each of which contains contributions from expert researchers in the field, and provides an authoritative and practical guide to the study of exRNA. This collection of methods and protocols will serve as a useful resource for those interested in this exciting and emerging field.

The first section provides an overview of the field. Chapter 1 starts with a concise and up-to-date review of exRNA research, whereas Chapter 2 provides an overview that guides the reader toward the use of appropriate protocols for isolation of exRNA, or extracellular vesicles and their associated RNA content. These chapters provide the context and background for subsequent chapters that describe methods and protocols for isolation of exRNA.

The second section focuses on approaches for the isolation of exRNA. Chapters 3 and 4 describe methods for isolation of exRNA and RNA associated with extracellular vesicles from cells in culture. An approach for the large-scale production of extracellular vesicles that provides greater exRNA yield is described in Chapter 4. An overview of standard approaches for the isolation of extracellular vesicles from body fluids such as serum, plasma, or bile is provided in Chapters 5 and 6. These methods could be adopted for use in other body fluids, but with modifications that depend on the nature, protein content, and composition of exRNA within each fluid. Chapters 7–9 provide more specialized and refined approaches for separation of extracellular vesicles such as cushioned density gradient ultracentrifugation, magnetic or affinity chromatography. These may be particularly useful for specific downstream applications and can be adapted for greater selectivity. Other than RNA present within extracellular vesicles, exRNA can be associated with lipoproteins or other proteins. Protocols for the isolation of such nonvesicular RNA are described in Chapters 10 and 11.

The third section outlines protocols for the detection and quantitation of exRNA. The extent to which RNA content within extracellular vesicles reflects either their cellular origin or underlying disease state will determine their potential application as biomarkers. The use of exRNA as disease biomarkers requires reliable methods for their detection and quantitation. The three chapters in this section discuss methods for the analysis of exRNA. Sensitivity of detection is a major challenge in the field of exRNA because approaches such as Northern blot or quantitative real-time PCR are often limited by the small amounts of exRNA present in body fluids or within extracellular vesicles. Chapters 12–14 outline approaches for the use of digital PCR, the optimization of approaches for preparation of libraries for next-generation sequencing, and the use of nanostring for detection and analysis of exRNA.

The last section describes approaches that can be useful for studies to evaluate potential therapeutic applications. Due to their important roles in intercellular communication, extracellular vesicles have been evaluated as carriers to deliver therapeutic agents across biological membranes. Chapters 15 and 16 outline methods for the use of extracellular vesicles to deliver therapeutic RNA molecules.

The range of topics covered in this book will be of interest to scientists and researchers, teachers and students, biotechnology companies and entrepreneurs interested in this rapidly emerging field of exRNA research. The sections are inter-related and are not just collections of independent protocols. Thus, the refinement of methods for isolation of vesicular or nonvesicular exRNA will complement the approaches for detection and quantitation. Likewise, the application of appropriate methods for isolation of extracellular vesicles will support approaches for their use in therapeutic applications. Nevertheless, individual nuances are also reflected within the protocols, in order to provide a useful guide.

In closing, we would like to thank all of the authors for their outstanding and valuable contributions, members of the NIH Common Fund Program on Extracellular RNA for their support and guidance, Caitlyn Foerst for her expert administrative assistance, and for all those involved in the production of the book. We hope that the reader will find this collection valuable and that the use of the methods and protocols within this book will further enhance the field of exRNA research.

Jacksonville, FL, USA   *Tushar Patel*

Contents

Contributors

ROGER ALEXANDER • *Pacific Northwest Diabetes Research Institute, Seattle, WA, USA*

NEIL ARONIN • *RNA Therapeutics Institute, University of Massachusetts Medical School, Worcester, MA, USA; Department of Medicine, University of Massachusetts Medical School, Worcester, MA, USA*

SAWEN BAKR • *Cardiovascular Research Center, Massachusetts General Hospital, Boston, MA, USA*

LEONORA BALAJ • *Department of Neurosurgery, Massachusetts General Hospital and Harvard Medical School, Boston, MA, USA*

DAVID BAXTER • *Institute for Systems Biology, Seattle, WA, USA*

VALENTIN X. BERDAH • *Department of Transplantion, Mayo Clinic, Jacksonville, FL, USA*

DAVID A. BORRELLI • *Department of Transplantion, Mayo Clinic, Jacksonville, FL, USA*

MARIKE BROEKMAN • *Department of Neurology, Massachusetts General Hospital and Harvard Medical School, Boston, MA, USA; Department of Neurosurgery, Brain Center Rudolf Magnus University Medical Center Utrecht, Utrecht, The Netherlands*

ALFONSO CAYOTA • *Functional Genomics Unit, Institut Pasteur de Montevideo, Montevideo, Uruguay; Department of Medicine, Faculty of Medicine, Universidad de la República, Montevideo, Uruguay*

LILIAN CRUZ • *Department of Neurology, Massachusetts General Hospital and Harvard Medical School, Boston, MA, USA*

KIRSTY M. DANIELSON • *Cardiovascular Research Center, Massachusetts General Hospital, Boston, MA, USA*

SAUMYA DAS • *Cardiovascular Research Center, Massachusetts General Hospital, Boston, MA, USA*

MARIE-CECILE DIDIOT • *RNA Therapeutics Institute, University of Massachusetts Medical School, Worcester, MA, USA; Department of Molecular Medicine, University of Massachusetts Medical School, Worcester, MA, USA*

SOPHIE A. DUSOSWA • *Department of Neurology, Massachusetts General Hospital and Harvard Medical School, Boston, MA, USA; Department of Molecular Cell Biology and Immunology, VU University Medical Center, Amsterdam, The Netherlands; Amsterdam Infection & Immunity Institute, VU University Medical Center, Amsterdam, The Netherlands; Cancer Center Amsterdam, VU University Medical Center, Amsterdam, The Netherlands*

ALTON ETHERIDGE • *Pacific Northwest Research Institute, Seattle, WA, USA*

JUSTYNA FILANT • *Department of Gynecologic Oncology and Reproductive Medicine, The University of Texas MD Anderson Cancer Center (MDACC), Houston, TX, USA*

DAVID GALAS • *Pacific Northwest Research Institute, Seattle, WA, USA*

ROOPALI GANDHI • *Department of Neurology, Center for Neurologic Diseases, Brigham and Women's Hospital, Harvard Medical School, Boston, MA, USA*

ALESSANDRA GURTNER • *Department of Neurosurgery, Massachusetts General Hospital and Harvard Medical School, Boston, MA, USA; Department of Life Sciences, University of Trieste, Trieste, Italy*

BENCE GYORGY • *Department of Neurology, Massachusetts General Hospital and Harvard Medical School, Boston, MA, USA*

REKA A. HARASZTI • *RNA Therapeutics Institute, University of Massachusetts Medical School, Worcester, MA, USA; Department of Molecular Medicine, University of Massachusetts Medical School, Worcester, MA, USA*

PETE HEINZELMAN • *Department of Neuroscience, Mayo Clinic-Jacksonville, Jacksonville, FL, USA*

KING YEUNG HONG • *Department of Surgery, University of California & VA Medical Center, San Francisco, CA, USA*

MICHELLE E. HUNG • *Interdisciplinary Biological Sciences Program, Northwestern University, Evanston, IL, USA*

ANASTASIA KHVOROVA • *RNA Therapeutics Institute, University of Massachusetts Medical School, Worcester, MA, USA; Department of Molecular Medicine, University of Massachusetts Medical School, Worcester, MA, USA*

ROY Y. KIM • *Department of Surgery, University of California & VA Medical Center, San Francisco, CA, USA*

LOUISE C. LAURENT • *Department of Reproductive Medicine, University of California, San Diego, La Jolla, CA, USA*

STEPHEN B. LENZINI • *Department of Chemical and Biological Engineering, Northwestern University, Evanston, IL, USA*

JOSHUA N. LEONARD • *Department of Chemical and Biological Engineering, Northwestern University, Evanston, IL, USA; Center for Synthetic Biology, Northwestern University, Evanston, IL, USA; Chemistry of Life Processes Institute, Northwestern University, Evanston, IL, USA; Member, Robert H. Lurie Comprehensive Cancer Center, Northwestern University, Evanston, IL, USA*

KANG LI • *Department of Surgery, University of California & VA Medical Center, San Francisco, CA, USA*

RISHABH LOHRAY • *Department of Transplantation, Mayo Clinic, Jacksonville, FL, USA*

FU SANG LUK • *Department of Surgery, University of California & VA Medical Center, San Francisco, CA, USA*

AKIKO MATSUDA • *Department of Transplantation, Mayo Clinic, Jacksonville, FL, USA; Department of Cancer Biology, Mayo Clinic, Jacksonville, FL, USA*

PARHAM NEJAD • *Department of Neurology, Center for Neurologic Diseases, Brigham and Women's Hospital, Harvard Medical School, Boston, MA, USA*

TUSHAR PATEL • *Department of Transplantion, Mayo Clinic, Jacksonville, FL, USA; Department of Cancer Biology, Mayo Clinic, Jacksonville, FL, USA*

ANU PAUL • *Department of Neurology, Center for Neurologic Diseases, Brigham and Women's Hospital, Harvard Medical School, Boston, MA, USA*

ROBERT L. RAFFAI • *Department of Surgery, University of California & VA Medical Center, San Francisco, CA, USA*

RODOSTHENIS S. RODOSTHENOUS • *Cardiovascular Division of the Massachusetts General Hospital and Harvard Medical School, Boston, MA, USA*

NOAH SADIK • *Department of Neurosurgery, Massachusetts General Hospital and Harvard Medical School, Boston, MA, USA*

ANE MIREN SALVADOR-GARICANO • *Cardiovascular Division of the Massachusetts General Hospital and Harvard Medical School, Boston, MA, USA*

NEHA SHUKLA • *Department of Transplantion, Mayo Clinic, Jacksonville, FL, USA*

BRIDGET SIMONSON • *Cardiovascular Research Center, Massachusetts General Hospital, Boston, MA, USA*

JULIA SMALL • *Department of Neurosurgery, Massachusetts General Hospital and Harvard Medical School, Boston, MA, USA*

THOMAS SEBASTIAAN VAN SOLINGE • *Department of Neurology, Massachusetts General Hospital and Harvard Medical School, Boston, MA, USA; NeuroDiscovery Center, Harvard Medical School, Boston, MA, USA; Department of Neurosurgery, VU University Medical Center, Amsterdam, The Netherlands*

ANIL K. SOOD • *Department of Gynecologic Oncology and Reproductive Medicine, The University of Texas MD Anderson Cancer Center (MDACC), Houston, TX, USA; Center for RNA Interference and Non-Coding RNAs, MDACC, Houston, TX, USA; Department of Cancer Biology, MDACC, Houston, TX, USA*

SRIMEENAKSHI SRINIVASAN • *Department of Reproductive Medicine, University of California, San Diego, La Jolla, CA, USA*

DEVIN M. STRANFORD • *Department of Chemical and Biological Engineering, Northwestern University, Evanston, IL, USA*

JUAN PABLO TOSAR • *Functional Genomics Unit, Institut Pasteur de Montevideo, Montevideo, Uruguay; Nuclear Research Center, Faculty of Science, Universidad de la República, Montevideo, Uruguay*

KAI WANG • *Institute for Systems Biology, Seattle, WA, USA*

ZHIYUN WEI • *Department of Neurology, Brigham and Women's Hospital and Harvard Medical School, Boston, MA, USA*

DAVID K. WONG • *Department of Surgery, University of California & VA Medical Center, San Francisco, CA, USA*

IRENE K. YAN • *Department of Transplantion, Mayo Clinic, Jacksonville, FL, USA*

XUAN ZHANG • *Department of Neurology, Massachusetts General Hospital, Harvard Medical School, Boston, MA, USA*

OLIVIA ZIEGLER • *Cardiovascular Division of the Massachusetts General Hospital and Harvard Medical School, Boston, MA, USA*

Chapter 1

Extracellular RNAs: A New Awareness of Old Perspectives

Noah Sadik, Lilian Cruz, Alessandra Gurtner, Rodosthenis S. Rodosthenous,
Sophie A. Dusoswa, Olivia Ziegler, Thomas Sebastiaan Van Solinge,
Zhiyun Wei, Ane Miren Salvador-Garicano, Bence Gyorgy,
Marike Broekman, and Leonora Balaj

Abstract

Extracellular RNA (exRNA) has recently expanded as a highly important area of study in biomarker discovery and cancer therapeutics. exRNA consists of diverse RNA subpopulations that are normally protected from degradation by incorporation into membranous vesicles or by lipid/protein association. They are found circulating in biofluids, and have proven highly promising for minimally invasive diagnostic and prognostic purposes, particularly in oncology. Recent work has made progress in our understanding of exRNAs—from their biogenesis, compartmentalization, and vesicle packaging to their various applications as biomarkers and therapeutics, as well as the new challenges that arise in isolation and purification for accurate and reproducible analysis. Here we review the most recent advancements in exRNA research.

Key words Extracellular vesicles, RNA, Exosomes, Microvesicles, Vesicle biogenesis, Biomarkers, Noncoding RNA

1 Background

exRNA has emerged as an important source of biological information that represents the dynamic processes that occur intra- and intercellularly, in real time. exRNAs are released in a variety of subpopulations that vary amongst cell lines and are isolated via differing protocols. Here we discuss the potential of exRNAs in unraveling a new understanding of information trafficking in cells as well as the challenges in analyzing them in an accurate and reproducible fashion.

Tushar Patel (ed.), *Extracellular RNA: Methods and Protocols*, Methods in Molecular Biology, vol. 1740,
https://doi.org/10.1007/978-1-4939-7652-2_1, © Springer Science+Business Media, LLC 2018

2   Biogenesis of exRNA and Role in Cell Biology

Most exRNA is protected from degradation by incorporation into membranous vesicles or association with lipids and/or proteins. Several subtypes of extracellular vesicles (EVs) have been described, including exosomes (<150 μm), microvesicles (200–500 μm), and oncosomes (1–10 μm) [1, 2]. Various biogenesis mechanisms are responsible for the formation of EVs. Whereas exosomes are shed through the multivesicular bodies of the endosomal pathway, microvesicles or ectosomes have been shown to bud off from the plasma membrane, and oncosomes can be released directly from tumor cell membranes. It is believed that the mechanism responsible for their formation influences their content, which consists of messenger RNA (mRNA), small noncoding (ncRNAs), DNA, proteins, and lipids. This content can be transferred to different cells and can mediate functional effects in these cells. Indeed, EVs have been shown to play a role in various biological processes, varying from establishing a body plan during development [3], to pathological processes as the formation of metastatic niches in cancer [4]. However, the extent to which RNA contents are responsible for these effects remains to be elucidated. EVs are generally regarded as a powerful source of biomarkers for various diseases, including glioblastoma [5–7], as they can be found in body fluids and their contents reflect the active status of their cells of origin (Fig. 1).

3   Compartments of exRNAs

exRNAs circulate in biofluids (e.g., blood, urine, saliva, cerebrospinal fluid, breast milk, follicular fluid) as part of different compartments, which protect them from degradation by RNAses [8]. Namely, exRNAs are either encapsulated in EVs such as exosomes and larger vesicles [5], or bound in complexes with proteins such as the Argonaute 2 (Ago2) and high-density lipoproteins (HDLs) [9, 10]. Recent studies have shown that the profiles of exRNAs by compartment is different. For instance, while EVs are abundant in microRNAs (miRNAs), other types of RNAs are also detected, including small nucleolar RNAs (snoRNAs), PIWI-interacting RNAs (piRNAs), long noncoding RNAs (lncRNAs), transfer RNAs (tRNAs) and tRNA fragments, YRNAs, ribosomal RNAs (rRNAs), mitochondrial RNAs, and protein-coding RNAs [11–13]. On the contrary, the cargo of HDL:RNA complexes consist mainly of noncoding RNAs such as miRNAs, tRNA fragments, ribosomal RNAs, snoRNAs, and lncRNAs, but no protein-coding RNAs [14]. Lastly, Ago2 has binding affinity for miRNAs only [9, 14, 15].

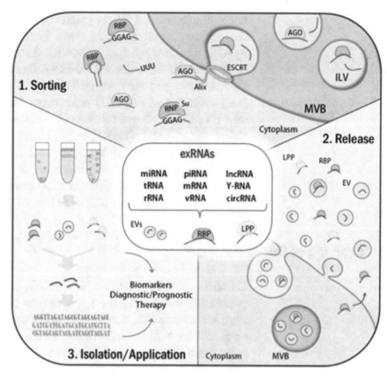

Fig. 1 Sorting, release, and isolation/application of exRNAs. As shown in the central panel, several types of RNAs and fragments of RNAs have been detected extracellularly associated with EVs, RBP, and/or lipoproteins (e.g., HDL). (*1*) *Sorting*: RNAs sorting mechanisms into EVs. RBPs can bind to RNAs by recognizing specific motifs, sequence or structure and target them into EVs. RNA modification such as uridylation (U) has shown to be enriched in EVs when compared to the intracellular content. Argonaute proteins (AGO) are canonical miRNAs binding partners and are related to miRNAs sorting into EVs by mechanism that may involve Alix, an ESCRT member. hnRNPA2B1, an RNP, when modified by SUMO (Su) recognizes certain motifs in miRNAs and regulates their sorting into EVs. (*2*) *Release*: ExRNAs are released by the cells combined to RBPs (e.g., AGO), lipoproteins (e.g., HDL), or EVs. (*3*) *Isolation/Application*: Extracellular RBPs, lipoproteins, and vesicles can be isolated by using different techniques, such as differential ultracentrifugation, density gradient or immunocapture, and the RNAs can be purified for further sequencing or functional assays. exRNAs sources (EVs, RBP, lipoproteins) and exRNAs detection could be used as biomarkers or potential therapies. *AGO:* argonaute, *EVs:* extracellular vesicles, *ESCRT:* endosomal sorting complex required for transport, *ILV:* intralumenal vesicle, *MVB:* multivesicular bodies, *RBP:* RNA-binding protein, *RNP:* ribonucleoprotein

4 Proposed Mechanisms of exRNA Packaging into EVs

Packaging of exRNAs in EVs is an active and orchestrated process that favors the sorting and enrichment of certain exRNAs in EVs, whereas it excludes others. To date, two major mechanisms have been characterized to regulate this process, an Ago2- and a chaperone-mediated mechanism. Recent studies have shown that Ago2 is a potent mediator of miRNAs sorting into EVs and that it can be regulated by the KRAS-MEK signaling pathway [16]. Other studies have shown that miRNAs with specific sequence motifs (i.e., GGAG and GGCU) were recognized and selectively sorted into EVs by the chaperone proteins heterogeneous nuclear ribonucleoprotein A2B1 (hnRNPA2B1) and RNA-interacting protein SYNCRIP [17]. In addition, the RNA-binding protein Y-box I (YBX-1) is suggested to be involved in the packaging of miRNAs and other exRNAs into EVs by recognizing secondary rather than primary RNA sequence motifs [18].

5 Overview of Extracellular mRNAs

Of all the subpopulations of exRNA, mRNA is one of the least abundant, accounting for a proportion of about 2% [19]. This low number of mRNA molecules poses the first major challenge in extracellular mRNA sequencing. Extracellular mRNA could be isolated from biological fluids such as blood, urine, saliva, or cerebrospinal fluid, or from in vitro cell culture supernatants. To date, RNA sequencing studies looking at extracellular mRNA focus on EV-associated mRNA. exRNA profiles, however, could vary when using different protocols for cell culture or methods for vesicle isolation [19, 20]. Since different subpopulations of exRNA vary in abundance between fractions after ultracentrifugation [20], EV isolation methods will clearly affect exRNA sequencing profiles. Furthermore, in cell cultures requiring fetal bovine serum (FBS), exRNA isolates are contaminated with FBS-derived exRNA, found in both the EV containing pellet and the supernatant after ultracentrifugation [20]. Up to 13% of FBS RNA reads can be mapped to the human or mouse genome, indicating that FBS-derived RNA significantly contributes to false-positive findings in both human and mouse exRNA sequencing studies [20]. Indeed, after re-analysis of publicly available exRNA sequencing datasets, in exosomes, roughly 2.6–17.2% of exRNA reads corresponded to bovine-specific transcripts [20]. For extracellular miRNA sequencing, the number of unique miRNAs had been shown to plateau at a sequencing depth of ten million reads [19]. For extracellular mRNA, however, optimal sequencing depth is unknown. Quantification of mRNA abundances requires normalization of their expression levels to well-established reference controls. Unfortunately, these controls have not yet been established for any of the exRNA subpopulations, including mRNA [19]. Additionally, for studies involving biomarker discovery for different disease conditions, a healthy control reference is currently lacking. Altogether, the field of extracellular mRNA sequencing faces considerable challenges, including the major concerns of low yield, FBS-derived mRNA contamination, and the lack of standardization of mRNA-seq library preparation.

6 Other Classes of exRNAs: microRNAs

miRNAs are small, noncoding post-transcriptional regulators of gene expression. They play important roles in diverse cellular processes, both in regulatory pathways and by acting as buffers to stochastic changes in transcription [21, 22]. It is estimated approximately 60% of all mRNAs are targeted by miRNAs [23]. miRNAs are highly processed; they are initially transcribed as components of long precursor transcripts, often many kilobases in length, called pri-miRNAs. These may be co-transcribed along with the mRNAs they regulate, or may be in distant locations of the DNA [24]. These pri-miRNAs form hairpin structures and are trimmed by the RNAse III, Drosha, to form a pre-miRNA that is exported from the nucleus in association with Exportin 5. When it enters the cytoplasm, its loop structure is cut by the endoribonuclease, Dicer. The mature miRNA, called the guide strand, forms one half of resulting RNA duplex, and is loaded into the miRNA silencing complex, miRISC, in association with the catalytically active component, Ago2 [25]. miRNAs suppress translation of mRNAs either by direct competitive blocking or by altering the stability of the target mRNA. This destabilization either occurs from shortening of the polyA tail or, if the miRNA has high complementarity with the target mRNA, Ago2 may directly cut the target [26–28]. miRNAs recognize their target mRNAs primarily through their seed sequences, a 6–8 nucleotide sequence near the 5′ end of the miRNA [29]. This region typically exhibits high complementarity with targets. In animals, the remainder of the miRNA does not require perfect complementarity to effectively suppress target mRNAs. Consequently, miRNAs are promiscuous regulators of many genes; each may act on dozens to hundreds of mRNAs [30]. Though miRNAs are abundant in the cytosol, they are also released into the extracellular environment either within vesicles or associated with low-density lipoproteins or other lipoproteins. As a consequence of this release, miRNAs are able to act on sites distant from their synthesis, are important mediators of cell-to-cell communication, and have demonstrated utility as biomarkers of both physiologic and pathologic processes [31–33].

6.1 Transfer RNAs

Transfer RNA (tRNA) is a 78–90 nucleotide RNA structure involved in the translation of mRNA to proteins, transporting amino acids to the ribosome where the anticodon of the tRNA binds to the complementary triplet mRNA codon and links the amino acids to form proteins [34]. However, an increasing amount of research shows that tRNA plays an important role in other cellular functions as well, influencing mRNA cleavage, inhibiting translation, and promoting morphological changes [35]. tRNA constitutes a large part of the RNAs found in exosomes, in larger proportions compared to other cellular RNAs [36–38]. This over-representation of tRNA has been observed in EVs shed by breast cells, bone marrow and adipose-mesenchymal stem cells, lung cells, semen, urine, and blood serum [37–40]. In contrast, EVs shed by melanoma cells appear to contain very little tRNA, while the proportion of tRNA in the microvesicles and apoptotic bodies shed by these cells is similar to that of the cellular cytoplasm [41]. The selection of tRNA found within an EV further indicates the discriminatory shedding of tRNA in EVs. One example was observed after the deep sequencing of EVs shed by mouse dendritic- and T cells: roughly seven times more reads of tRNA-Lys-AAA were observed in RNA derived from EVs compared to RNA recovered from intracellular space [36]. Aside from full-length tRNAs, EVs appear to harbor tRNA fragments (tRFs) in high concentrations [36, 37]. The exact mechanism of function of tRFs is unclear to date, but they are suspected to be involved in specific regulatory pathways [42]. For instance, the half of the tRNA-Gly containing the 5′ end suppresses protein synthesis, while smaller tRNA fragment inhibit translation nonspecifically [43, 44]. Similar increases of 5′ end tRNA halves in EVs have been recorded in breast, HeLa, and lung cell lines [37]. The reasons for which tRNAs and tRNA halves are concentrated in EVs, and whether those components are functionally transferred to cytosols of other cells remain to be known.

6.2 PIWI-Interacting RNAs

Among the small RNAs that guide gene regulation, piRNAs are the largest class of small ncRNA molecules expressed in animal cells, having prospects of hundreds of thousands of distinct piRNA species [45]. piRNAs are about 22–30-nt-long molecules that protect germ line cells from transposons, mobile genetic elements that threaten an organism's genome. They guide PIWI-clade Ago proteins to complementary RNAs derived from transposable elements, where the PIWI proteins cleave transposon RNA, leading to silencing [46]. piRNAs are generated independently of Dicer from single-stranded precursors with the help of two RNP complexes [47]. Germ granules, specifically, pi-bodies, and a germ line analog of processing bodies, piP-bodies, are the cytoplasmic compartments where PIWI pathway components assemble [48]. Little is known about the extracellular presence of piRNAs. Although they had not been previously known to be widely present in biofluids, a 2016 study by Freedman et al. identified 144 small RNAs in circulation that mapped to piRNAs [45]. To distinguish piRNAs from other exRNAs, the study included two distinct reverse transcriptase experiments showing that piRNA RT-qPCR analyses were specific to piRNA 3′ modifications. Abundance of most piRNA species in B cells, neutrophils, peripheral mononuclear cells, platelets, and T cells were found to be nonsignificantly different from their abundances on plasma. However, B cells, neutrophils, platelets, and T cells had significant numbers of upregulated piRNA species as compared with plasma, while a majority of piRNA species were shown to be upregulated in red blood cells as compared with plasma. Interestingly, most piRNAs in exosomes were either not significantly different from downregulated as compared with plasma [45]. We do not yet know why piRNAs end up in EVs and whether they are functionally transferred to other cells.

6.2.1   YRNAs

YRNA is a very conserved class of small noncoding RNA [49] ranging from 84 to 113 nucleotides long in humans. It is highly abundant in cells, having a greater presence than tRNA and U6 snRNA. In extracellular fractions, including MVs, exosomes and RNPs, YRNAs have lower abundances than in cells, but are still more abundant than most miRNAs. Despite their high abundance levels, only four species exist in humans: Y1, Y3, Y4, and Y5. Furthermore, YRNAs have not been studied comprehensively, with less than 100 publications in PubMed. The lower stem domain of YRNAs was found to play a role in RNA quality control and degradation of misfolded RNAs by recruiting chaperone Ro60 and exoribonuclease PNPase [50]. The upper stem domain may participate in the initiation of chromosomal DNA replication [51]. YRNAs can be further processed to YRNA fragments, with the majority of modifications at the 5′ end. Although initially mistakenly thought of as miRNAs, these YRNA fragments are now known to be distinct entities. Their biogenesis is independent of Dicer, and they do not bind to Ago2 [52]. Functionally, YRNA fragments do not seem to silence target expression in a miRNA-like manner, as evidenced by a luciferase reporter assay [53]. The biological functions of YRNA fragments have not been clarified yet, but recent studies reported that they might be involved in cell damaging [54] and histone mRNA processing [55]. Interestingly, although YRNA fragments are less abundant than their full-length versions in cellular RNA, fragment abundance is higher than full-length abundance in extracellular fractions, and especially in RNP fractions where fragments contribute to approximately 20% of non-rRNA small RNA [56]. Further studies focusing on their biogenesis, secretion, and functions offer exciting new directions in RNA biology.

6.3   Other Noncoding RNAs

Apart from mRNAs, miRNAs, piRNAs, tRNAs, and YRNAs that are widely abundant in both cellular and extracellular spaces, the advent of next-generation sequencing revealed a broad spectrum of additional ncRNAs that are present in the acellular portions of biofluids [57, 58]. In the range of newly detectable exRNA, a significant expression of lncRNAs, small nuclear RNAs (snRNAs), snoRNAs, and circular RNAs (circRNAs) were detected [19, 23, 58, 59]. lncRNAs are any nonprotein-coding RNAs with a length >200 nucleotides that lack a long open reading frame and/or do not show codon conservation. Since their relatively low evolutionary preservation and their low level of expression, some posited that they represented only "transcriptional noise" and/or redundant transcripts with no biological significance [60]. However, it is now clear that the lack of primary sequence conservation in lncRNAs does not indicate lack of function [61, 62]. The expression of TUC339, for example, a lncRNA that is selectively released in EV from hepatocellular cancer cells, has a foundational role in modulating tumor cell behavior [63]. snRNAs were found to be localized in EVs. Although their intracellular functions are noted and mainly related to RNA splicing, methylation, and pseudouridylation [64], their role in extracellular spaces is still poorly known. Appaiah, H.N. and colleagues, in 2011, identified U6, small nuclear RNA, that is upregulated in the sera of cancer patients [65]. Sequence analysis showed also that there were diverse collections of snoRNAs in human plasma-derived EV RNAs, among which C1orf213, LINC00324, and LOC388692 were the most abundant [58]. Despite the limited information available regarding their expression and function in human tissues, new examinations using an ion proton system for plasma of 40 individuals revealed that snoRNAs appear to primarily guide chemical modifications of other RNAs, managing alternative splicing and gene silencing [45]. In addition to linear RNA molecules described above, a specific type of ncRNA, circRNA, is generated from pre-mRNA with a back-splice mechanism, that connects the 3' end and 5' end of a transcript's precursor to form a circle [66]. A circular structure makes circRNA more resistant to exonucleases than other types of RNAs, preventing from the characteristic degradation and digestion of molecules in extracellular spaces [66, 67]. Its hypothetical function involves downregulation of miRNAs by sequestering complementary miRNAs like a sponge [59].

7 Challenges in Isolating exRNA Subpopulations

Optimization of methods to isolate high-purity exRNA subpopulations and measuring quantity and integrity is a current technical challenge in exRNA research. The most studied exRNA subpopulation comprises the RNAs found in EVs. However, many biological effects associated with EV-RNA could also be caused by the presence of other RNA-containing components [15, 68], such as ribonucleoprotein complexes, viral particles, and lipoproteins (e.g., HDL and LDL). The source of these non-EV RNA-carriers could be the EV's biological sample of origin or the fetal bovine serum in cell culture media [69, 70]. The yield and purity of EVs depend on the EVs isolation method, which consequently, defines the quantity and quality of EV-RNA [71–73]. Because current highly sensitive molecular techniques can detect small amounts of components in EV preparations, co-purification of non-EV contaminants generates a significant artifact for further RNA analysis [74–76].

EV isolation techniques are based on different biophysical properties of EVs, such as density, shape, size, and surface proteins and therefore enrich for different subpopulations of vesicles, although none of the methods recover a pure material containing only EVs [77]. These methods include differential ultracentrifugation, density gradient centrifugation, chromatography, filtration, polymer-based precipitation, and immunoaffinity. Ultracentrifugation is the most widely used method; however, the EV pellet can be contaminated with protein aggregates and viruses [78]. Density gradient centrifugation can be used in combination with ultracentrifugation to isolate highly purified EVs from other extracellular source of RNAs; however, this results in low yields. Lipoprotein may be co-isolated when the starting sample is plasma or serum [79]. Size exclusion chromatography consists of a size-based separation in a column. It promotes high EV recovery and removes most soluble contaminants, but other particles with similar pore-cutoff size may co-elute with the EVs [80]. Filtration can concentrate EVs and may remove soluble components, but similarly sized particles can contaminate the sample [81]. Precipitation techniques have high EV recovery rates, but also precipitate non-EV components [82]. Immunoaffinity uses antibodies against proteins found in EVs; thus, it can be used to isolate EV subpopulations. However, non-EV proteins might also be recovered. Indeed, the specific details of these purification procedures can differ significantly between different groups causing variability in the recovery of EVs, resulting in weaker detection of RNA in EVs and detection of RNA-carrying contaminants [79]. Several alternative techniques, many as commercially available kits, have been developed to improve EV purification, such as antibody-coated magnetic beads, affinity beads, novel precipitation (e.g., ExoQuick and Total Exosome Isolation) and filtration kits (e.g., PureExo), membrane affinity spin columns (e.g., ExoEasy), and microfluidics-based techniques (e.g., ExoChip) [83–88]. Particularly, ExoEasy kit allows recovering of both EVs and other soluble RNA-carriers separately [85]. Moreover, a combination of techniques has been described for purification of non-EV exRNA sources [9, 14, 89]. Despite the rapid growth of the exRNA research in the last few years, the field still needs standardized methods, both for isolation and characterization of exRNA subpopulations to enable successful exRNA applications as biomarkers and therapeutics.

8   exRNA as Biomarkers

exRNAs are contained and relatively stable within circulating vesicles in most biological fluids [90]. Among exRNAs, both miRNAs and piRNAs are the most highly enriched RNA species within extracellular vesicles, with a lower representation of long noncoding RNA, fragments of tRNA, YRNA and mRNA, among others [19]. exRNA-containing vesicles are present in most biofluids, consisting of a mixture of vesicles of different origin; either cells present in body fluids (e.g., blood [91], breast milk [92], and follicular fluid [93]) or cells contouring the space irrigated by body fluids (e.g., saliva, urine) [94]. Considering the advantage of easily collecting exRNA from biofluids in a noninvasive manner, many studies indicate that, in addition to having an important function in intercellular communication, exRNA could also be used as potential biomarkers as indicators of normal biological processes, as candidates for early stage diagnostic in patients at risk, and also as predictors of pathology recurrence after treatment. There is substantial evidence indicating that exRNA can be used both for diagnostic and prognostic purposes in the oncology field [95]. For instance, tumor-derived exRNA (e.g., hTERT mRNA and miR-141) can be detected in blood of prostate cancer patients, correlating with tumor size and malignancy [70, 96]. Among the tumors in the digestive system, a variety of serum miRNA is found expressed differentially in hepatocellular carcinoma and chronic hepatitis. Additionally, exRNA in saliva is reported to be associated with pancreatic [97] and esophageal cancer [98]. As an additional example of exRNA used as biomarkers in the oncology field, miR-21, which is elevated in glioblastoma patients, has been shown to discriminate this from healthy patients [99]. Similarly, in cardiovascular disease, myocardial specific circulating miRNAs are significantly elevated in advanced heart failure, correlating with a concomitant increase in classical peptide biomarkers of myocardial damage like cardiac troponin I [100]. Furthermore, lncRNA could be considered as independent predictors of pathological cardiac remodeling and diastolic dysfunction in patients diagnosed with diabetes type 2 [101]. In addition to the oncology and cardiovascular fields indicated above, exRNA has also been described as potential biomarkers for pathological conditions in the nephrology [102] and neurology [95] fields, as well as in pregnancy [103, 104].

9   exRNA as Therapeutics for Cancer

To facilitate therapeutic delivery, exRNA can be packaged in stable natural carriers. Most studies have focused on using EVs as carriers for miRNA, siRNA, or other nucleic acids. Packaging anticancer nucleic acids in tumor-targeting EVs offers a novel method for cancer therapy. For example, Ohno et al. demonstrated that expressing GE11 peptide on the surface of EVs targets EGFR-positive tumor cells and that the delivery of a tumor suppressor miRNA, let-7a was able to inhibit breast cancer development in vivo [105]. In another study, microvesicle-encapsulated TGFβ1 siRNA was shown to inhibit murine sarcoma growth in vitro and in vivo [106]. The authors demonstrated that siRNA was associated with argonaute complexes in MVs, suggesting that MV packaged exRNA is stable and readily assembled for downstream gene silencing, as argonaute proteins are part of the RISC complex [107]. Mesenchymal stem cells (MSC) are being increasingly utilized as the source of EVs due to accessibility and therapeutic potency [108]. MSC-derived EVs were shown to be able to deliver anticancer small RNA in several cancer models, including osteosarcoma [110], hepatocellular carcinoma [110], bladder cancer [111], and glioblastoma multiforme. In these studies, miRNA or anti-miRNA-loaded EVs were able to inhibit tumor growth and migration, induce apoptosis, and render tumor cells more sensitive to chemotherapeutic agents. Although EVs are robust carriers of small RNA species, larger RNA species (such as mRNA) were also shown to be incorporated into these structures. The mRNA of a suicide gene was packaged in EVs that were able to inhibit tumor growth in a schwannoma model after the addition of the suicide drug [112]. However, it can be challenging to differentiate between the effects of mRNA or protein made from this mRNA in the producer cells. Taken together, the above examples suggest that exRNA packaged in EVs has therapeutic potential and once scalability and manufacturing of these complex drug carriers are established, they have an enormous potential in anticancer drug therapy.

10 Conclusion

As our knowledge of exRNA continues to rapidly expand, we are bound to learn more about vaguely understood exRNA subpopulations and their potential applications in medical diagnostics and novel therapeutic pipelines. As a lack of optimized and standardized methods to isolate high-purity exRNA subpopulations still challenges the field, future efforts must be made for the unification of these processes. Nevertheless, the promising field of exRNA research may soon revolutionize the way we look at cancer and related diagnostics in terms of quality, cost, efficiency, uniformity, and real-time analytic capabilities, as well as the future of targeted medicine in cancer therapy.

Acknowledgements

B.G. is an Edward R. and Anne G. Lefler Center Postdoctoral Fellow. The authors declare no conflicts of interest.

References

1. Di Vizio D et al (2012) Large oncosomes in human prostate cancer tissues and in the circulation of mice with metastatic disease. Am J Pathol 181(5):1573–1584

2. Minciacchi VR, Freeman MR, Di Vizio D (2015) Extracellular vesicles in cancer: exosomes, microvesicles and the emerging role of large oncosomes. Semin Cell Dev Biol 40:41–51

3. Yanez-Mo M et al (2015) Biological properties of extracellular vesicles and their physiological functions. J Extracell Vesicles 4:27066

4. Costa-Silva B et al (2015) Pancreatic cancer exosomes initiate pre-metastatic niche formation in the liver. Nat Cell Biol 17(6):816–826

5. Skog J et al (2008) Glioblastoma microvesicles transport RNA and proteins that promote tumour growth and provide diagnostic biomarkers. Nat Cell Biol 10(12):1470–1476

6. Chen WW et al (2013) BEAMing and droplet digital PCR analysis of mutant IDH1 mRNA in glioma patient serum and cerebrospinal fluid extracellular vesicles. Mol Ther Nucleic Acids 2:e109

7. Balaj L et al (2011) Tumour microvesicles contain retrotransposon elements and amplified oncogene sequences. Nat Commun 2:180

8. Lasser C et al (2011) Human saliva, plasma and breast milk exosomes contain RNA: uptake by macrophages. J Transl Med 9:9

9. Turchinovich A et al (2011) Characterization of extracellular circulating microRNA. Nucleic Acids Res 39(16):7223–7233

10. Vickers KC et al (2011) MicroRNAs are transported in plasma and delivered to recipient cells by high-density lipoproteins. Nat Cell Biol 13(4):423–433

11. Crescitelli R et al (2013) Distinct RNA profiles in subpopulations of extracellular vesicles: apoptotic bodies, microvesicles and exosomes. J Extracell Vesicles 2

12. Lasser C et al (2017) Two distinct extracellular RNA signatures released by a single cell type identified by microarray and next-generation sequencing. RNA Biol 14(1):58–72

13. Bellingham SA, Coleman BM, Hill AF (2012) Small RNA deep sequencing reveals a distinct miRNA signature released in exosomes from prion-infected neuronal cells. Nucleic Acids Res 40(21):10937–10949

14. Michell DL et al (2016) Isolation of high-density lipoproteins for non-coding small RNA quantification. J Vis Exp (117)

15. Arroyo JD et al (2011) Argonaute2 complexes carry a population of circulating microRNAs independent of vesicles in human plasma. Proc Natl Acad Sci U S A 108(12):5003–5008

16. Cha DJ et al (2015) KRAS-dependent sorting of miRNA to exosomes. Elife 4:e07197

17. Villarroya-Beltri C et al (2013) Sumoylated hnRNPA2B1 controls the sorting of miRNAs into exosomes through binding to specific motifs. Nat Commun 4:2980

18. Shurtleff MJ et al (2016) Y-box protein 1 is required to sort microRNAs into exosomes in cells and in a cell-free reaction. Elife 5

19. Yuan T et al (2016) Plasma extracellular RNA profiles in healthy and cancer patients. Sci Rep 6:19413

20. Wei Z et al (2016) Fetal bovine serum RNA interferes with the cell culture derived extracellular RNA. Sci Rep 6:31175

21. Musilova K, Mraz M (2015) MicroRNAs in B-cell lymphomas: how a complex biology gets more complex. Leukemia 29(5):1004–1017

22. Ebert MS, Sharp PA (2012) Roles for microRNAs in conferring robustness to biological processes. Cell 149(3):515–524

23. Friedman RC et al (2009) Most mammalian mRNAs are conserved targets of microRNAs. Genome Res 19(1):92–105

24. Rodriguez A et al (2004) Identification of mammalian microRNA host genes and transcription units. Genome Res 14(10A):1902–1910

25. Pratt AJ, MacRae IJ (2009) The RNA-induced silencing complex: a versatile gene-silencing machine. J Biol Chem 284(27):17897–17901

26. Filipowicz W, Bhattacharyya SN, Sonenberg N (2008) Mechanisms of post-transcriptional regulation by microRNAs: are the answers in sight? Nat Rev Genet 9(2):102–114

27. Eulalio A et al (2009) Deadenylation is a widespread effect of miRNA regulation. RNA 15(1):21–32

28. Hutvagner G, Zamore PD (2002) A microRNA in a multiple-turnover RNAi enzyme complex. Science 297(5589):2056–2060

29. Nielsen CB et al (2007) Determinants of targeting by endogenous and exogenous microRNAs and siRNAs. RNA 13(11):1894–1910

30. Bartel DP (2009) MicroRNAs: target recognition and regulatory functions. Cell 136(2):215–233

31. Chen X et al (2012) Secreted microRNAs: a new form of intercellular communication. Trends Cell Biol 22(3):125–132

32. Vickers KC, Remaley AT (2012) Lipid-based carriers of microRNAs and intercellular communication. Curr Opin Lipidol 23(2):91–97

33. Melman YF et al (2015) Circulating MicroRNA-30d is associated with response to cardiac resynchronization therapy in heart failure and regulates cardiomyocyte apoptosis: a translational pilot study. Circulation 131(25):2202–2216

34. Sharp SJ et al (1985) Structure and transcription of eukaryotic tRNA genes. CRC Crit Rev Biochem 19(2):107–144

35. Hurto RL (2011) Unexpected functions of tRNA and tRNA processing enzymes. Adv Exp Med Biol 722:137–155

36. Nolte-'t Hoen EN et al (2012) Deep sequencing of RNA from immune cell-derived vesicles uncovers the selective incorporation of small non-coding RNA biotypes with potential regulatory functions. Nucleic Acids Res 40(18):9272–9285

37. Tosar JP et al (2015) Assessment of small RNA sorting into different extracellular fractions revealed by high-throughput sequencing of breast cell lines. Nucleic Acids Res 43(11):5601–5616

38. Baglio SR et al (2015) Human bone marrow- and adipose-mesenchymal stem cells secrete exosomes enriched in distinctive miRNA and tRNA species. Stem Cell Res Ther 6:127

39. Li M et al (2014) Analysis of the RNA content of the exosomes derived from blood serum and urine and its potential as biomarkers. Philos Trans R Soc Lond Ser B Biol Sci 369(1652)

40. Vojtech L et al (2014) Exosomes in human semen carry a distinctive repertoire of small non-coding RNAs with potential regulatory functions. Nucleic Acids Res 42(11):7290–7304

41. Lunavat TR et al (2015) Small RNA deep sequencing discriminates subsets of extracellular vesicles released by melanoma cells—evidence of unique microRNA cargos. RNA Biol 12(8):810–823

42. Lee YS et al (2009) A novel class of small RNAs: tRNA-derived RNA fragments (tRFs). Genes Dev 23(22):2639–2649

43. Ivanov P et al (2011) Angiogenin-induced tRNA fragments inhibit translation initiation. Mol Cell 43(4):613–623

44. Sobala A, Hutvagner G (2013) Small RNAs derived from the 5′ end of tRNA can inhibit protein translation in human cells. RNA Biol 10(4):553–563

45. Freedman JE et al (2016) Diverse human extracellular RNAs are widely detected in human plasma. Nat Commun 7:11106

46. Meister G (2013) Argonaute proteins: functional insights and emerging roles. Nat Rev Genet 14(7):447–459

47. Hayashi R et al (2016) Genetic and mechanistic diversity of piRNA 3′-end formation. Nature 539(7630):588–592

48. Chuma S, Pillai RS (2009) Retrotransposon silencing by piRNAs: ping-pong players mark their sub-cellular boundaries. PLoS Genet 5(12):e1000770

49. Kowalski MP, Krude T (2015) Functional roles of non-coding Y RNAs. Int J Biochem Cell Biol 66:20–29

50. Chen X et al (2013) An RNA degradation machine sculpted by Ro autoantigen and noncoding RNA. Cell 153(1):166–177

51. Krude T et al (2009) Y RNA functions at the initiation step of mammalian chromosomal DNA replication. J Cell Sci 122(Pt 16):2836–2845

52. Nicolas FE et al (2012) Biogenesis of Y RNA-derived small RNAs is independent of the microRNA pathway. FEBS Lett 586(8):1226–1230

53. Meiri E et al (2010) Discovery of microRNAs and other small RNAs in solid tumors. Nucleic Acids Res 38(18):6234–6246

54. Chakrabortty SK et al (2015) Extracellular vesicle-mediated transfer of processed and functional RNY5 RNA. RNA 21(11):1966–1979

55. Kohn M et al (2015) The Y3** ncRNA promotes the 3′ end processing of histone mRNAs. Genes Dev 29(19):1998–2003

56. Wei Z, Batagov AO, Schinelli S, Wang J, Wang Y, El Fatimy R, Rabinovsky R, Balaj L, Chen CC, Hochberg F, Carter B, Breakefield XO, Krichevsky AM (2017) Coding and noncoding landscape of extracellular RNA released by human glioma stem cells. Nat Commun 8(1):1145

57. Yeri A et al (2017) Total extracellular small RNA profiles from plasma, saliva, and urine of healthy subjects. Sci Rep 7:44061

58. Huang X et al (2013) Characterization of human plasma-derived exosomal RNAs by deep sequencing. BMC Genomics 14:319

59. Hansen TB et al (2013) Natural RNA circles function as efficient microRNA sponges. Nature 495(7441):384–388

60. Morris KV, Mattick JS (2014) The rise of regulatory RNA. Nat Rev Genet 15(6):423–437

61. Smith MA et al (2013) Widespread purifying selection on RNA structure in mammals. Nucleic Acids Res 41(17):8220–8236

62. Johnsson P et al (2014) Evolutionary conservation of long non-coding RNAs; sequence, structure, function. Biochim Biophys Acta 1840(3):1063–1071

63. Kogure T et al (2013) Extracellular vesicle-mediated transfer of a novel long noncoding RNA TUC339: a mechanism of intercellular signaling in human hepatocellular cancer. Genes Cancer 4(7–8):261–272

64. Maxwell ES, Fournier MJ (1995) The small nucleolar RNAs. Annu Rev Biochem 64:897–934

65. Appaiah HN et al (2011) Persistent upregulation of U6:SNORD44 small RNA ratio in the serum of breast cancer patients. Breast Cancer Res 13(5):R86

66. Chen LL (2016) The biogenesis and emerging roles of circular RNAs. Nat Rev Mol Cell Biol 17(4):205–211

67. Memczak S et al (2013) Circular RNAs are a large class of animal RNAs with regulatory potency. Nature 495(7441):333–338

68. Turchinovich A, Burwinkel B (2012) Distinct AGO1 and AGO2 associated miRNA profiles in human cells and blood plasma. RNA Biol 9(8):1066–1075

69. Shelke GV et al (2014) Importance of exosome depletion protocols to eliminate functional and RNA-containing extracellular vesicles from fetal bovine serum. J Extracell Vesicles 3

70. Mitchell PS et al (2008) Circulating microRNAs as stable blood-based markers for cancer detection. Proc Natl Acad Sci U S A 105(30):10513–10518

71. Brunet-Vega A et al (2015) Variability in microRNA recovery from plasma: comparison of five commercial kits. Anal Biochem 488:28–35

72. Li X, Mauro M, Williams Z (2015) Comparison of plasma extracellular RNA isolation kits reveals kit-dependent biases. Biotechniques 59(1):13–17

73. Royo F et al (2016) Different EV enrichment methods suitable for clinical settings yield different subpopulations of urinary extracellular vesicles from human samples. J Extracell Vesicles 5:29497

74. Van Deun J et al (2014) The impact of disparate isolation methods for extracellular vesicles on downstream RNA profiling. J Extracell Vesicles 3

75. Laurent LC et al (2015) Meeting report: discussions and preliminary findings on extracellular RNA measurement methods from laboratories in the NIH Extracellular RNA Communication Consortium. J Extracell Vesicles 4:26533

76. Tanriverdi K et al (2016) Comparison of RNA isolation and associated methods for extracellular RNA detection by high-throughput quantitative polymerase chain reaction. Anal Biochem 501:66–74

77. Gardiner C et al (2016) Techniques used for the isolation and characterization of extracellular vesicles: results of a worldwide survey. J Extracell Vesicles 5:32945

78. Jeppesen DK et al (2014) Comparative analysis of discrete exosome fractions obtained by differential centrifugation. J Extracell Vesicles 3:25011

79. Yuana Y et al (2014) Co-isolation of extracellular vesicles and high-density lipoproteins using density gradient ultracentrifugation. J Extracell Vesicles 3

80. Boing AN et al (2014) Single-step isolation of extracellular vesicles by size-exclusion chromatography. J Extracell Vesicles 3

81. Vergauwen G et al (2017) Confounding factors of ultrafiltration and protein analysis in extracellular vesicle research. Sci Rep 7(1):2704

82. Gamez-Valero A et al (2016) Size-exclusion chromatography-based isolation minimally alters extracellular vesicles' characteristics compared to precipitating agents. Sci Rep 6:33641

83. Kanwar SS et al (2014) Microfluidic device (ExoChip) for on-chip isolation, quantification and characterization of circulating exosomes. Lab Chip 14(11):1891–1900

84. Balaj L et al (2015) Heparin affinity purification of extracellular vesicles. Sci Rep 5:10266

85. Enderle D et al (2015) Characterization of RNA from exosomes and other extracellular vesicles isolated by a novel spin column-based method. PLoS One 10(8):e0136133

86. Gallart-Palau X et al (2015) Extracellular vesicles are rapidly purified from human plasma by PRotein Organic Solvent PRecipitation (PROSPR). Sci Rep 5:14664

87. Shih CL et al (2016) Development of a magnetic bead-based method for the collection of circulating extracellular vesicles. New Biotechnol 33(1):116–122

88. Puhka M et al (2017) KeepEX, a simple dilution protocol for improving extracellular vesicle yields from urine. Eur J Pharm Sci 98:30–39

89. Turchinovich A, Weiz L, Burwinkel B (2013) Isolation of circulating microRNA associated with RNA-binding protein. Methods Mol Biol 1024:97–107

90. Thery C, Ostrowski M, Segura E (2009) Membrane vesicles as conveyors of immune responses. Nat Rev Immunol 9(8):581–593

91. Schipper HM et al (2007) MicroRNA expression in Alzheimer blood mononuclear cells. Gene Regul Syst Bio 1:263–274

92. Karlsson O et al (2016) Detection of long non-coding RNAs in human breastmilk extracellular vesicles: implications for early child development. Epigenetics:0

93. Machtinger R et al (2017) Extracellular microRNAs in follicular fluid and their potential association with oocyte fertilization and embryo quality: an exploratory study. J Assist Reprod Genet 34(4):525–533

94. Dear JW, Street JM, Bailey MA (2013) Urinary exosomes: a reservoir for biomarker discovery and potential mediators of intrarenal signalling. Proteomics 13(10–11):1572–1580

95. Quinn JF et al (2015) Extracellular RNAs: development as biomarkers of human disease. J Extracell Vesicles 4:27495

96. March-Villalba JA et al (2012) Cell-free circulating plasma hTERT mRNA is a useful marker for prostate cancer diagnosis and is associated with poor prognosis tumor characteristics. PLoS One 7(8):e43470

97. Xie Z et al (2013) Salivary microRNAs as promising biomarkers for detection of esophageal cancer. PLoS One 8(4):e57502

98. Xie Z et al (2015) Salivary microRNAs show potential as a noninvasive biomarker for detecting resectable pancreatic cancer. Cancer Prev Res (Phila) 8(2):165–173

99. Akers JC et al (2013) MiR-21 in the extracellular vesicles (EVs) of cerebrospinal fluid (CSF): a platform for glioblastoma biomarker development. PLoS One 8(10):e78115

100. Akat KM et al (2014) Comparative RNA-sequencing analysis of myocardial and circulating small RNAs in human heart failure and their utility as biomarkers. Proc Natl Acad Sci U S A 111(30):11151–11156

101. de Gonzalo-Calvo D et al (2016) Circulating long-non coding RNAs as biomarkers of left ventricular diastolic function and remodelling in patients with well-controlled type 2 diabetes. Sci Rep 6:37354

102. Ben-Dov IZ et al (2016) Cell and microvesicle urine microRNA deep sequencing profiles from healthy individuals: observations with potential impact on biomarker studies. PLoS One 11(1):e0147249

103. Rodosthenous RS, Burris HH, Sanders AP, Just AC, Dereix AE, Svensson K, Solano M, Téllez-Rojo MM, Wright RO, Baccarelli AA (2017) Second trimester extracellular microRNAs in maternal blood and fetal growth: an exploratory study. Epigenetics 12(9):804–810

104. Tsochandaridis M, Nasca L, Toga C, Levy-Mozziconacci A (2015) Circulating MicroRNAs as clinical biomarkers in the predictions of pregnancy complications. BioMed Res Int 2015:294954

105. Ohno S et al (2013) Systemically injected exosomes targeted to EGFR deliver antitumor microRNA to breast cancer cells. Mol Ther 21(1):185–191

106. Zhang Y et al (2014) Microvesicle-mediated delivery of transforming growth factor beta1 siRNA for the suppression of tumor growth in mice. Biomaterials 35(14):4390–4400

107. Jinek M, Doudna JA (2009) A three-dimensional view of the molecular machinery of RNA interference. Nature 457(7228): 405–412

108. Lai RC, Yeo RW, Lim SK (2015) Mesenchymal stem cell exosomes. Semin Cell Dev Biol 40:82–88

109. Shimbo K et al (2014) Exosome-formed synthetic microRNA-143 is transferred to osteosarcoma cells and inhibits their migration. Biochem Biophys Res Commun 445(2):381–387

110. Lou G et al (2015) Exosomes derived from miR-122-modified adipose tissue-derived MSCs increase chemosensitivity of hepatocellular carcinoma. J Hematol Oncol 8:122

111. Greco KA et al (2016) PLK-1 silencing in bladder cancer by siRNA delivered with exosomes. Urology 91:241.e1–241.e7

112. Mizrak A et al (2013) Genetically engineered microvesicles carrying suicide mRNA/protein inhibit schwannoma tumor growth. Mol Ther 21(1):101–108

Chapter 2

Overview of Protocols for Studying Extracellular RNA and Extracellular Vesicles

Julia Small, Roger Alexander, and Leonora Balaj

Abstract

Understanding the role of extracellular RNA (exRNA) has emerged as an exciting avenue for biomarker, therapeutic, as well as basic cell–cell communication applications and discoveries. Multiple protocols, kits, and procedures have been developed in the last decade to allow fractionation as well as isolation of sub-populations of macromolecules of interest found in biofluids. Here, we introduce the protocols decision tree developed by the Extracellular RNA Communication Consortium and available on their website (exRNA portal), and compare all methods currently available to the exRNA field and report pros and cons for each platform.

Key words Extracellular RNA, Exosomes, Biomarkers, Ribonuclear particles, Kits, Protocols

The Extracellular RNA Communication Consortium (ERCC) has spent the last several years developing protocols for the isolation and characterization of extracellular RNA (exRNA). The main goal of this work has been to ensure that the protocols are robust enough to minimize variation in methodology and results across labs. The amount of exRNA found in biofluids is very low, limited by both our isolation and detection/sequencing technologies. Therefore, it is vital to further progress this kind of cross-validation work in order to better understand the natural function of exRNAs and their applications as disease biomarkers and therapeutic agents.

For researchers who have just begun studying extracellular RNA, including the extracellular vesicles in which they are often encapsulated by, the ERCC has developed a protocols decision tree to help select the appropriate set of protocols for isolating EVs and exRNA from the biofluids of interest. The protocols decision tree [1] is available on the ERCC's website, the exRNA Portal [2]. While some of the protocols in the decision tree have been developed by ERCC researchers, many of the protocols consist of previously published methods that have been modified by ERCC members during the course of their experiments and are being periodically updated. In particular, the decision tree makes refer-

Tushar Patel (ed.), *Extracellular RNA: Methods and Protocols*, Methods in Molecular Biology, vol. 1740, https://doi.org/10.1007/978-1-4939-7652-2_2, © Springer Science+Business Media, LLC 2018

ence mostly to protocols published on *Nature*'s Protocol Exchange (NPE) repository. Initial versions were released on NPE in December 2015, and a second version of most protocols were release on NPE in June 2017. The major difference between the first and second versions of the protocols is an increase in the initial amount of biofluid processed, from 200 to 500 μL. We found that the larger input volume led to higher levels of RNA isolation and therefore more uniformity in results across labs. The decision tree will continue to be updated with new protocol versions as they become available.

Here, we introduce the ERCC protocols decision tree and discuss some of the nuanced differences between classes of EV isolation methods, highlighting methods that have existed in the field for some time.

There are several methods and commercial kits available to isolate extracellular vesicles (EVs) and extracellular RNA (exRNA) from human biofluids. Multiple studies have reported on a variety of these methods, but to date there is not one method or kit that suits all studies. The type of biofluid, the sample volume, and the fraction of exRNAs of interest are some of the criteria used to determine what method should be used for a particular study. Here, we have compiled a list of methods and kits most widely reported in literature for isolation of EVs, exRNAs, or other components of biofluids. Broadly speaking, all methods can be classified into five categories (*see* Table 1), the most widely used being ultracentrifugation.

Drawbacks of ultracentrifugation include the need for expensive instrumentation (ultracentrifuges and rotors) and the belief that the EV population after ultracentrifugation will be contaminated with cell-free DNA and proteins. Depending on the speed and time of ultracentrifugation, some ribonucleoprotein (RNP) and lipoprotein (LPP) complexes may also sediment. After ultracentrifugation, some researchers further purify the EV population using density gradients or size exclusion chromatography. Sucrose gradients have been used widely for several years but are being replaced more recently by iodixanol (OptiPrep) gradients. This is because some groups have reported that sucrose may inhibit the biological effects of EVs, while EVs prepared with OptiPrep better retain their biological activity.

Size exclusion chromatography is also widely used and is suitable for fractionation of sedimented EVs, as well as unprocessed biofluids. Recently, Izon introduced a commercial kit to speed up this method, with relatively good results. Size exclusion chromatography yields a very clean population of EVs with the drawback being loss of EVs during the multistep purification process.

The first commercial EV isolation kit (Exoquick™) was launched on the market about 7 years ago, and is based on the principle of polyethylene glycol/sodium chloride precipitation,

Table 1
Methods of extracellular vesicle purification and extracellular RNA isolation

	EV isolation	Manufacturer	Application	Reference
Ultracentrifugation	Step 1. 300–3000 × g 5–30 min	The most widely used protocol	Removes cells	[3]
	Step 2. 10,000–20,000 × g for 30 min[a]		Removes debris	
	Step 3. 100,000–167,000 × g for 1–18 h		Pellets EVs	
Sample purification	Sucrose gradient	Lab-developed method	All biofluids	[3]
	OptiPrep gradient	Sigma-Aldrich	All biofluids	[4]
	Size exclusion chromatography	Lab-developed method	All biofluids	[5]
	qEV	Izon	All biofluids	[4]
Precipitation	ExoQuick™	System Biosciences	Serum, plasma, cell culture media	[6]
	Total exosome isolation	Life Technologies Inc.	Serum, plasma, cell culture media	[7]
	Exosome RNA isolation	Norgen Biotek Corp.	Serum, plasma, urine	[8]
	miRCURY™ exosome kit	Exiqon	Serum, plasma, urine, CSF, cell culture media	[9]
Filtration	Sequential fractionation using different size filters	Krichevsky Lab[1]	Cell culture media	[10]
	ExoMir™	BIOO Scientific	All biofluids	[11]
Affinity purification	ExoCap™ (CD9, CD63, CD81, EpCAM)	JSR Micro	Serum, plasma, cell culture media	MBL International
	Microfluidics Immunoaffinity	Irimia Lab	Serum, plasma	[12]
	Micro nuclear magnetic resonance (μNMR)	Weissleder Lab	Serum, ascites	[13]
	Heparin beads	Lab-developed method	Serum, plasma, cell culture media	[14]
	exoRNeasy	Qiagen	Serum, plasma, cell culture media	[15]
	PureExo[R][b]	101Bio	All biofluids	[16]
	Exo-spin™[c]	Cell Guidance System	Serum, plasma	[4]
	ME[TE] exosome kit	New England Peptide	Serum, plasma	[17]

[a]This step is omitted by several research groups
[b]Filtration first, then affinity to proprietary matrix
[c]Precipitation first, then affinity to proprietary matrix

which has long been used for concentration of viruses. Since that time, several other kits using a precipitation strategy were launched by other manufacturers. Each of these kits (SBI, Life Technologies, Norgen Biotek, and Exiqon) has slightly different proprietary approaches to EV precipitation. Drawbacks to EV precipitation kits include coprecipitation of other unwanted molecules found in the biofluids and the difficulty of isolating EVs from large volumes of starting material. Ultrafiltration (e.g., using Millipore Amicon filters) is often used by researchers to concentrate large volumes, either before or after EV purification.

Filtration-based methods which isolate specific size ranges of EVs can also be performed using commercially available devices. In addition, several kits and protocols for affinity purification have been developed by biotechnology companies and academic research laboratories. Antibody-based affinity methods (ExoCap, Microfluids, μNMR) and heparin-coated agarose or magnetic beads have been shown to bind subpopulations of EVs from cell culture media, plasma, and serum efficiently. Another affinity kit, the ME[TE] kit, includes a proprietary peptide that, according to the manufacturer, binds to heat-shock proteins found on the surface of the plasma membrane, suggesting a possible method to enrich EVs with high levels of heat-shock proteins. All of these methods yield a pure sample of EVs and can be scaled up, although scale-up costs can be significant, particularly in the case of antibody-based methods. These methods are limited to isolating a subset of EVs that express a specific antigen. For researchers who are interested in targeting a specific population of EVs that displays one of these antigens, this may be a good option. However, at this point, for most cases, the biology is unclear on the diversity of EVs released by cells. Therefore, one antibody, or a pool of three to four antibodies, may not isolate all relevant EVs present in the sample.

ExoRNeasy isolates EVs based on their affinity to a proprietary membrane. ERCC members using this kit have reported that it can efficiently separate EVs (they bind to the membrane with high affinity) from other exRNA-containing particles, such as RNP complexes, which can be collected in the flow-through. Thus, this kit offers the extra advantage of efficiently separating EVs from RNP complexes. The exoRNeasy/exoEasy kit can yield a pure EV population from a volume as low as 200 L or as high as 4 mL of plasma or serum with one loading per column, and up to 100 mL of cultured media per column by loading the column 3–4 times. Larger volumes require loading multiple filters.

Two kits available on the market are based on a two-step procedure where the sample is first either filtered (e.g., PureExo) or concentrated (e.g., Exo-Spin) and then resuspended and allowed to bind to proprietary beads. Intact EVs are then eluted in phosphate-buffered saline (PBS) and can be used for a variety of downstream assays. These kits do not offer feasible approaches to scale up to larger volumes.

Many other combinations and variations on these methods have also been reported in literature, and this list is not meant to comprehensively encompass all reports in the field. It is a simple overview of the major classes of EV and RNA isolation methods currently available.

References

1. http://tinyurl.com/exRNA-protocols/
2. http://exRNA.org/resources/protocols/
3. Thery C, Amigorena S, Raposo G, Clayton A (2006) Isolation and characterization of exosomes from cell culture supernatants and biological fluids. Curr Protoc Cell Biol. Chapter 3, Unit 3.22
4. Lobb RJ et al (2015) Optimized exosome isolation protocol for cell culture supernatant and human plasma. J Extracell Vesicles 4. https://doi.org/10.3402/jev.v4.27031
5. Boing AN et al (2014) Single-step isolation of extracellular vesicles by size-exclusion chromatography. J Extracell Vesicles 3. https://doi.org/10.3402/jev.v3.23430
6. Taylor DD, Zacharias W, Gercel-Taylor C (2011) Exosome isolation for proteomic analyses and RNA profiling. Methods Mol Biol 728:235–246
7. Vlassov AV, Magdaleno S, Setterquist R, Conrad R (2012) Exosomes: current knowledge of their composition, biological functions, and diagnostic and therapeutic potentials. Biochim Biophys Acta Gen Subj 1820:940–948
8. Muralidharan J et al (2017) Extracellular microRNA signature in chronic kidney disease. Am J Physiol Renal Physiol 312:F982–F991
9. Lasser C, Eldh M, Lotvall J (2012) Isolation and characterization of RNA-containing exosomes. J Vis Exp (59):e3037. https://doi.org/10.3791/3037
10. Zhiyun Wei, Arsen O. Batagov, Sergio Schinelli, Jintu Wang, Yang Wang, Rachid El Fatimy, Rosalia Rabinovsky, Leonora Balaj, Clark C. Chen, Fred Hochberg, Bob Carter, Xandra O. Breakefield, Anna M. Krichevsky, (2017) Coding and noncoding landscape of extracellular RNA released by human glioma stem cells. Nature Communications 8 (1)
11. Bryant RJ et al (2012) Changes in circulating microRNA levels associated with prostate cancer. Br J Cancer 106:768–774
12. Chen C et al (2010) Microfluidic isolation and transcriptome analysis of serum microvesicles. Lab Chip 10:505–511
13. Shao H et al (2012) Protein typing of circulating microvesicles allows real-time monitoring of glioblastoma therapy. Nat Med 18:1835–1840
14. Balaj L et al (2015) Heparin affinity purification of extracellular vesicles. Sci Rep 5:10266
15. Enderle D et al (2015) Characterization of RNA from exosomes and other extracellular vesicles isolated by a novel spin column-based method. PLoS One 10:e0136133
16. Osteikoetxea X, Nemeth A, Sodar BW, Vukman KV, Buzas EI (2016) Extracellular vesicles in cardiovascular disease: are they Jedi or Sith? J Physiol 594:2881–2894
17. Ghosh A et al (2014) Rapid isolation of extracellular vesicles from cell culture and biological fluids using a synthetic peptide with specific affinity for heat shock proteins. PLoS One 9:e110443

Chapter 3

Extracellular RNA Isolation from Cell Culture Supernatant

Sawen Bakr, Bridget Simonson, Kirsty M. Danielson, and Saumya Das

Abstract

Extracellular RNAs are emerging as novel biomarkers and mediators of intercellular communication. Various methods to isolate RNA from biofluids and cell culture supernatants have been previously used by investigators. Here, we describe several standardized protocols for the isolation of RNAs from cell culture supernatants that utilize commercially available kits and reagents.

   Key words RNA isolation, Extracellular vesicles, Extracellular RNA, Cell culture supernatant, Plasma

1 Introduction

Extracellular RNAs (exRNAs) have recently come to prominence as a novel class of biomarker for numerous diseases including cancers, cardiovascular disease, and autoimmune disorders [1, 2]. They represent a heterogeneous group of RNAs including microRNA, piwi-interacting RNA, small nucleolar RNA, Y-RNAs, and t-RNA fragments [3]. exRNAs are stable in body fluids and cell culture supernatant (CCS), and may be packaged in extracellular vesicles (EVs), or bound to proteins or lipoprotein complexes [4, 5]. In addition to their role as biomarkers for prognosis and detection of disease, exRNAs have numerous functional roles in normal physiology, pathology of diseases, and cell–cell communication [6].

One of the greatest challenges to studying exRNAs is the development of reliable and consistent RNA isolation methods. exRNA isolation is challenging for several reasons including: (1) low RNA amounts present in biofluids and CCS; (2) effective separation and isolation of RNA from stabilizing complexes (EVs, proteins, or lipoproteins); (3) potential degradation of the RNA by RNAses; and (4) the presence of inhibitors in plasma or CCS that decrease RNA yield or inhibit downstream applications. This chapter describes methods for the isolation of exRNA from CCS that have been successfully employed in conjunction with downstream applications including qRT-PCR, microarrays, and RNA sequencing.

Tushar Patel (ed.), *Extracellular RNA: Methods and Protocols*, Methods in Molecular Biology, vol. 1740,
https://doi.org/10.1007/978-1-4939-7652-2_3, © Springer Science+Business Media, LLC 2018

2 Materials

2.1 Pre-Clearing CCS Supernatant

1. 50 mL falcon tubes.
2. Steriflip, 0.22 μm PES membrane EMD Millipore.

2.2 Differential Ultracentrifugation

1. 14 × 89 mm open top Beckman Coulter Polypropylene tubes.
2. RNAse–DNAse-free Phosphate-buffered saline, pH 7.4.

2.3 Density Gradient Ultracentrifugation

1. 14 × 89 mm open top Beckman Coulter Polypropylene tubes.
2. 25 x 89 mm open top Beckman Coulter Polyallomer tubes.
3. *Sucrose/Tris solution*: Dissolve 0.25 M sucrose in 10 mM Tris buffer and pH to 7.5, and pass through a 0.22 μm filter.
4. *Gradient buffers*: Dilute Optiprep (Iodixanol 60% w/v) with 0.25 M sucrose/20 mM Tris (pH 7.5) to make the following concentrations: 40%, 20%, 10%, and 5%. Filter the solutions through a 0.22 μm filter.

2.4 Differential Filtration

1. RNAse–DNAse-free Phosphate-buffered saline, pH 7.4.
2. 50 mL falcon conical centrifuge tubes.
3. AU-15 millipore filter, 10 kDa MWCO EMD Millipore UFC901024.

2.5 Qiagen miRNeasy Kit

1. Qiagen miRNeasy micro kit—217084.
2. Chloroform.
3. 70% ethanol.
4. 100% ethanol.
5. RNase-free water.
6. 1.5 mL microfuge tubes.
7. Phase lock gel tubes, 2 mL.

2.6 Qiagen ExoRNeasy Maxi Kit

1. Qiagen ExoRNeasy Maxi kit—77064.
2. Chloroform.
3. 100% ethanol.
4. Phase lock gel tubes, 2 mL.
5. Microfuge tubes, 1.5 mL.

2.7 System Bioscience Exoquick Seramir Tissue Culture Kit

1. Exoquick Seramir tissue culture kit—Systems Biosciences, RA800-TC1.
2. 100% ethanol.
3. Microfuge tubes 1.5 mL.

2.8 Equipment	1. Microfuge.
	2. Vortex.
	3. SW 41 Ti rotor.
	4. SW 32 Ti rotor.
	5. Beckman L8-M Ultracentrifuge.
	6. Eppendorf 5417R Centrifuge.

3 Methods

3.1 General Considerations (See Also Note 1)

Following harvesting of the CCS, we pre-clear the material to remove cellular debris within 30 min. Following this step, the researcher has to decide on whether they want to analyze exRNA in the total CCS, or focus on the EV fraction (*see* **Note 1**). As has been noted, exRNAs may be present in EVs, lipoprotein fractions or even bound to RNA binding proteins. Hence, the exact protocol followed will depend on the questions being posed by the investigator. Care needs to be taken to work in an RNAse-free environment (*see* **Note 2**), and the particular conditions for cell culture has to be determined for each type of cell line or primary cell culture (*see* **Notes 3–6**). Here, we describe the protocols for direct isolation of exRNAs from CCS (*see* Subheadings 3.7 and 3.8) or from enriched EVs (Subheadings 3.3–3.5). A schematic for the experimental flow is provided in Fig. 1.

There are several different methods available for the isolation or enrichment of EVs from CCS. These include:

1. *Ultracentrifugation*: Protocol is cheap and easy, but purity of the EV fraction is suboptimal due to coprecipitation of other particles such as lipoproteins, protein complexes, and cellular organelles released from damaged cells. These components may also interfere with downstream assays.

2. *Sucrose or iodixanol-based density gradients*: While in our experience this results in the purest EV fractions that work in functional and other downstream assays (such as RNAseq or qRT-PCR), the protocol is time-consuming and not amenable to high-throughput processing. The yield of exRNA is lower, and there is a limit on the input volume (based on the size of ultracentrifuge tubes). To process larger volumes, it is possible to first isolate EVs by ultracentrifugation (as above), and then further purify the fractions by density gradient fractionation.

3. *Precipitation methods using commercially available kits*: There are different reagents to precipitate EVs from CCS, but the purity of EVs using these reagents are the lowest of the methods described due to coprecipitation of other aggregates and particles; consequently, the yield of material is higher [7].

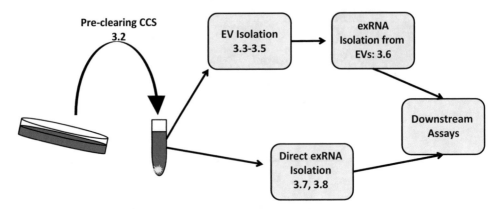

Fig. 1 Schematic for experimental flow for CCS exRNA Isolation

Here, we describe the use of the Exoquick reagent in conjunction with the Seramir Tissue Culture Kit; for the reasons stated above, we consider this direct exRNA isolation from CCS rather than selective isolation of RNAs from the EV fraction.

4. *Selective Filtration*: Using a filter for size selection of particles in CCS is easy and amenable to high-throughput; however, this method does not remove other particles and aggregates and can also lead to shearing of larger vesicles and contamination of the supposed EV fraction with fragments and contents of these sheared vesicles.

3.2 Pre-Clearing CCM Supernatant

Following harvesting of CCS, the supernatant should be precleared within 30 min to remove cellular debris. This step should be completed prior to either direct isolation of CCS exRNAs (*see* Subheadings 3.7 and 3.8) or EV enrichment prior to RNA isolation (*see* Subheadings 3.3–3.5). A schematic of the flow for direct isolation of exRNA from CCS, or isolation of exRNA from EVs derived from the CCS is shown in Fig. 1.

1. Harvest cell culture medium from 80% confluent cells (*see* **Note 6**) grown in serum-free medium for at least 24 h (*see* **Note 5**).

2. Transfer 5–10 mL of cell culture media from the Petri dish to an RNAse-free tube (15 mL Greiner Tubes) and centrifuge at 500–1000 × *g* for 10 min.

3. Transfer supernatant to a clean RNAse-free tube, avoiding any debris collected at the bottom of the tube, and centrifuge at 2000 × *g* for 10 min (we use the Eppendorf 5810R Centrifuge).

4. Transfer supernatant to a clean tube, again avoiding debris at the bottom of the tube, and pass through a 0.22 μm PES Steriflip membrane.

5. Proceed with RNA isolation or freeze media at −80 °C for later use (*see* **Note 7**).

6. Pre-cleared CCS can then be used for direct RNA isolation (*see* Subheadings 3.7 and 3.8) or can be processed for EV enrichment by one of the various methods noted below (Subheadings 3.3–3.5) prior to RNA isolation step (Subheading 3.6). This schema is demonstrated in Fig. 1.

3.3 Isolation of EVs by Ultracentrifugation

1. Use the desired volume of pre-cleared CCS (Subheading 3.2), we typically use 4–5 mL, and dilute to the top of the tube with sterile RNAse-free PBS. *Note*: ultracentrifuge tubes should be filled to close to the top to avoid collapse during centrifugation.

2. Centrifuge the pre-cleared supernatant at $100,000 \times g$ at 4 °C for 4 h.

3. Discard the supernatant and gently wash the pellet with 1 mL sterile RNAse-free PBS buffer, being careful to avoid dislodging the pellet.

4. Repeat **step 3** two additional times.

5. Resuspend the pellet with 1 mL sterile PBS and ultracentrifuge at $100,000 \times g$ at 4 °C for 120 min.

6. Discard the supernatant and resuspend the pellet in 200–500 µL of sterile RNAse-free PBS.

7. Proceed to RNA isolation (Subheading 3.6), further purify EVs by density gradient centrifugation (Subheading 3.4), or freeze the resuspension at −80 °C until required.

3.4 Iodixanol/ Tris-Sucrose Density Gradient (See Note 8)

1. Making density gradients: Pipette in each 14 × 89 mm tube the following dilutions in layers, starting with the highest concentration at the bottom (*see* **Note 9**). Add 1 mL CCS directly on top of the gradient; alternatively take the resuspension from ultracentrifugation of CCS (Subheading 3.3), add PBS to increase the volume to 1 mL and layer on the top of the gradient. In our experience, there is not enough material isolated from 1 mL of CCS to measure exRNAs in a meaningful manner although 1 mL of biofluids such as plasma has been successfully used in our laboratory for isolation of EVs to use in downstream assays. We therefore recommend using the resuspension from ultracentrifugation to add on top of the gradient.

   Volumes for the 14 × 89 mm tubes (from bottom of tube to top):

   - 2.5 mL 40%.
   - 2.5 mL 20%.
   - 2.5 mL 10%.
   - 1.5 mL 5%.
   - 1 mL sample for total volume of 10 mL.

2. Weigh the ultracentrifuge tubes to be within 0.01 g of each other. NB: it is critical that ultracentrifuges are correctly balanced prior to use to avoid damage to the rotor. Weights can be balanced by adding RNAse-free PBS buffer to the lighter tubes.

3. Load the tubes on the swinging bucket rotor SW41 Ti and run the centrifuge at $100,000 \times g$ for 18 h at 4 °C. In our laboratory, this is run on the Beckman L8-M Ultracentrifuge.

4. At the end of the centrifugation, there will be 12 fractions of 833 μL each in the centrifuge tube. The majority of exosomes are found in fraction 7, but other extracellular vesicles, such as microvesicles, are found in surrounding fractions (fractions 6–10). Depending on your targeted vesicle group, one or multiple fractions may be carefully pipetted out for further use.

5. Carefully pipette the desired fractions into a clean 25 × 89 mm polyallomer tube (30 mL tubes).

6. Centrifuge at $100,000 \times g$ for 2 h at 4 °C in the SW32 Ti rotor.

7. Wash the pellet very gently with 500 μL PBS.

8. Pipette and briefly vortex to resuspend the pellet in 200–500 μL RNAse-free PBS. Proceed to RNA isolation using the miRNeasy micro kit or store at −80 °C.

3.5 Millipore Membrane Filters

1. Use the pre-cleared CCS.

2. Before adding the filtered pre-cleared supernatant to an AU-15 filter, equilibrate an AU-15 filter with 2 mL of PBS. Then centrifuge the AU-15 filter at $3000–3500 \times g$ for 10 min in a swinging bucket rotor.

3. Carefully remove the PBS from the bottom of the filter and collection tube and discard solution.

4. Add 4 mL of the filtered pre-cleared supernatant to the AU-15 filter and centrifuge at $3000–3500 \times g$ for 30–50 min. This should result in about 500 μL of sample remaining in the upper chamber.

5. Discard the flow through and add 14 mL of PBS to the filter by gently pipetting. Mix by pipetting and centrifuge at $3000–3500 \times g$ for an additional 30–50 min until 200–500 μL of sample are left in the upper chamber.

6. Collect the concentrated sample from the upper chamber of the filter device. The sample can now be used for exRNA isolation using the Qiagen miRNeasy micro kit (*see* Subheading 3.6).

3.6 Qiagen miRNeasy Micro Kit (See Note 10)

1. Transfer EVs isolated from using any of the methods described in Subheadings 3.3–3.5 into a 1.5 mL microcentrifuge tube.

2. Add 5× volume of QIAzol Lysis Reagent and vortex gently for 5 s.

3. Prepare the PLG tubes by spinning for 30 s at 16,000 × g.

4. Add the sample from **step 2** to PLG tube (if necessary, split sample into two PLG tubes) and add the same volume of chloroform as the initial sample. In our case, the EVs are generally suspended in 200 μL, in which case we use 1 mL of QIAzol reagent and 200 μL of chloroform.

5. Shake (do not vortex) vigorously for 15 s.

6. Incubate for 3 min at room temperature.

7. Centrifuge the samples for 15 min at 12,000 × g at 4 °C.

8. Carefully transfer the upper aqueous phase to a new microcentrifuge tube without disrupting the organic layer or interface. You can pool the aqueous fractions here if they were split at **step 4**.

9. Measure the volume of this fraction, add 1.5× volume of 100% ethanol and mix gently but thoroughly.

10. Immediately load up to 700 μL of sample to an assembled MiniElute spin column, including any precipitate that may have formed, and spin for 15 s at 1000 × g at RT.

11. Discard flow through and repeat **step 10** until all the sample has been processed through the filter.

12. Wash the column by adding 700 μL Buffer RWT to the spin column and centrifuging at 8000 × g for 15 s at RT.

13. Discard the flow through.

14. Then wash the spin column by adding 500 μL Buffer RPE and centrifuging at 8000 × g for 15 s at RT.

15. Add 500 μL fresh 80% ethanol to the RNeasy MiniElute spin column and centrifuge at ≥8000 × g for 2 min at RT.

16. Discard the collection tube and flow through and transfer the spin column to a new 2 mL collection tube.

17. Open the lid of the spin column and centrifuge at full speed for 5 min to dry the membrane, discard the collection tube and flow through.

18. Transfer the spin column to a new 1.5 mL collection tube, and add 30 μL of RNase-free water. It is important to add the small volume of the water directly to the center of the spin column membrane without touching the membrane.

19. Centrifuge for 1 min at 100 × g followed by 1 min at full speed to elute the RNA. RNA can be used for the downstream assays such as qRT-PCR or RNAseq. Quantities of RNA depend on cell type and culture conditions.

Methods for Direct exRNA Isolation from CCS

3.7 ExoRNeasy Maxi Kit

1. This method uses the pre-cleared CCS (without subsequent processing to isolate EVs) to isolate exRNA.

2. Use the pre-cleared supernatant from Subheadings 3.2.

3. Transfer 4 mL of the filtered supernatant to a new 15 mL falcon tube.

4. Add 4 mL of XBP buffer to the 4 mL supernatant and mix gently by inverting for five times.

5. Transfer the supernatant/XBP mix to the exoEasy maxi spin column assembled in a collection tube.

6. Centrifuge at $500 \times g$ for 1 min at room temperature, discard the flow through in the collection tube.

7. Add 10 mL of XWP buffer into the exoEasy maxi spin column, then centrifuge at $3000–3500 \times g$ for 5 min at RT.

8. Transfer the exoEasy spin column into a new collection tube leaving the flow through behind.

9. Add 700 μL of Qiazol Lysis Reagent into the exoEasy spin column, then centrifuge at $3000–3500 \times g$ for 5 min.

10. Prepare the Phase Lock Tubes by centrifuging them at $16,000 \times g$ for 30 s.

11. Transfer the flow through from the exoEasy spin column (**step 9**) into the prepared Phase Lock Tubes and vortex the sample for 5 s.

12. Incubate at room temperature for 5 min.

13. Now add 90 μL chloroform to the sample and shake vigorously for 15 s. It is important to mix by shaking and not vortexing at this step.

14. Following incubation for 2 min at room temperature, centrifuge PLT with sample for 15 min at $12,000 \times g$ at 4 °C.

15. Carefully transfer the upper aqueous phase to a new microcentrifuge tube without disrupting the interface.

16. Add twice the volume (of the aqueous sample) of 100% ethanol to the sample and mix by pipetting up and down (do not vortex).

17. Pipet 650 μL of the mixture in the tube to the MinElute spin column.

18. Following centrifugation for 15 s at $1000 \times g$ at room temperature, discard flow through.

19. Repeat the **steps 22** and **23** until all the sample has been processed through the MinElute spin column.

20. For washing the MinElute spin column add 700 μL of RWT buffer in the MinElute spin column, following centrifugation for 15 s at $8000 \times g$ at room temperature.

21. After discarding the flow through from **step 20**, add 500 mL of the RPE buffer in the column, and centrifuge for 15 s at $8000 \times g$ at room temperature.

22. Discard the flow through.

23. Conduct an additional wash with 500 mL of the RPE buffer in the column, followed by centrifugation for 2 min at $\geq 8000 \times g$ at room temperature and discard the flow through.

24. Transfer the MinElute spin column into a new 2 mL collection tube.

25. Following centrifugation, open the lid of the column during the centrifugation and centrifuge at full speed for 5 min to dry the membrane.

26. Discard the collection tube with the flow through.

27. Transfer the spin column to a new 1,5 mL collection tube.

28. Add 14 µL of RNase-free water to the center of MinElute spin column and centrifuge for 1 min at $100 \times g$ followed by 1 min at full speed to elute the RNA. This can be used for downstream assays.

3.8 Exoquick SeraMir Tissue Culture Kit

1. Use the pre-cleared supernatant from Subheading 3.2.

2. Add 0.8 mL of Exoquick-TC buffer, then mix gently by inverting the tube three times.

3. Incubate the sample at 4 °C for 16 h.

4. Centrifuge at 13,000 rpm ($17,949 \times g$) for 2 min, discard the supernatant, and keep the exosome pellet. Note that the pellet may be hard to visualize.

5. Mix 350 µL lysis buffer to the sample by vortexing for 15 s. Incubate the sample for 5 min.

6. Add 200 µL of 100% ethanol and vortex the sample for 10 s.

7. Transfer the sample to the provided spin column, centrifuge at 13,000 rpm ($17,949 \times g$) for 1 min and discard the flow through.

8. Wash the column by adding 400 µL of wash buffer, followed by centrifugation at 13,000 rpm ($17,949 \times g$) for 1 min. Discard the flow through in the collection tube and repeat this step one more time.

9. Discard the flow through, then centrifuge for 2 min at 13,000 rpm ($17,949 \times g$) to dry the column.

10. Transfer the spin column to a new collection tube, and add 30 µL RNase-free water or Elution buffer to the center of the membrane.

11. Centrifuge for 2 min at $425 \times g$ followed by 1 min at 13,000 rpm on the Eppendorf 5417R centrifuge ($17,949 \times g$).

12. Collect the eluate and proceed to downstream assays or store at −80 °C.

4   Notes

1. There are several considerations that should be made prior to isolating exRNA. Firstly, it should be decided whether total RNA is required or a sub-compartment of exRNA, (e.g., EV-associated RNA). Methods for both total and EV RNA isolations are provided within this chapter. While the direct isolation kits (Subheadings 3.7 and 3.8) were designed to first precipitate "exosomes," we believe that the precipitating reagents bring down not only EVs (of all sizes), but also other types of aggregates and particles. Protocols to specifically isolate lipoprotein-coupled exRNAs are not addressed in this chapter.

2. Work should always be conducted in an RNAse-free environment. RNAses are ubiquitous; therefore, it is extremely critical to remove RNAses from surfaces and equipment before use and to use RNAse-free plastic ware and barrier pipette tips.

3. exRNA is released from cultured cells both at baseline and in response to stimuli [8]. To date, it appears that all cell types release exRNA; however, different cell types may release different amounts of exRNA and EVs. Furthermore, stimulation of cells can increase exRNA and EV production. For example, in cultured cardiomyocytes, ethanol added to the buffer to achieve concentrations of 21.7 and 65.1 mM can increase EV production [9]; and mechanical stretch can increase the release of miR-30d into the CCS [5]. Depending on the cell type being studied, the user may need to optimize conditions for optimal release of exRNAs.

4. Due to cell type and treatment differences, the volume of CCS required to detect exRNAs will vary between experiments. A starting volume of 5 mL CCS should be sufficient for most experiments but may require further optimization.

5. Another important consideration for CCS experiments is the content of the cell culture medium. Serum supplements such as fetal bovine serum (FBS) contain endogenous EVs (and thus RNA), which can confound experiments. If FBS is required for culturing conditions, prolonged ultracentrifugation ($100,000 \times g$ for 24 h) or an immunoaffinity method using antibodies against antigens on the EVs may be required to remove endogenous EVs in the FBS [10]. However, recent work suggests that even these methods are not entirely successful in removing exogenous EVs and exRNAs from media that contains FBS [11].

6. Cell density can also affect EV and exRNA release from cultured cells. Some studies have shown that high cell density results in decreased release of EVs [12]. One possible explanation

could be that at higher density, cells may preferentially shunt cellular pathways for release of EVs to intracellular trafficking pathways [13, 14].

7. Following pre-clearing, if not immediately using the sample, it is recommended to freeze large batches of CCS in multiple aliquots to avoid repeat freeze-thaw cycles.

8. The density gradient centrifugation method described here provides the "purest" EV fraction, but there is no evidence that this completely removes contaminating lipoproteins or protein aggregates.

9. When creating the layers for density gradient centrifugation, it is very important to pipet each layer very carefully to ensure that the dilutions don't intermix. Distinct layers should be visible after pipetting.

10. The EVs isolated in Subheadings 3.3–3.5 can be subjected to RNA isolation by various different methods and kits. We have described the Qiagen miRNeasy kit that we use for this application in our laboratory; however, other kits such as the miRVana PARIS isolation kit can also be used. We would suggest that individual users test these kits to assess the best yield under their conditions.

References

1. Redzic JS, Balaj L, van der Vos KE, Breakefield XO (2014) Extracellular RNA mediates and marks cancer progression. Semin Cancer Biol 28:14–23

2. Quinn JF, Patel T, Wong D, Das S, Freedman JE, Laurent LC et al (2015) Extracellular RNAs: development as biomarkers of human disease. J Extracell Vesicles 4:27495. https://doi.org/10.3402/jev.v4.27495

3. Schonrock N, Harvey RP, Mattick JS (2012) Long noncoding RNAs in cardiac development and pathophysiology. Circ Res 111(10):1349–1362

4. Etheridge A, Lee I, Hood L, Galas D, Wang K (2011) Extracellular microRNA: a new source of biomarkers. Mutat Res 717(1–2):85–90

5. Melman YF, Shah R, Danielson K, Xiao J, Simonson B, Barth A et al (2015) Circulating MicroRNA-30d is associated with response to cardiac resynchronization therapy in heart failure and regulates cardiomyocyte apoptosis: a translational pilot study. Circulation 131(25):2202–2216

6. Quesenberry PJ, Aliotta J, Deregibus MC, Camussi G (2015) Role of extracellular RNA-carrying vesicles in cell differentiation and repro-gramming. Stem Cell Res Ther 6:153. https://doi.org/10.1186/s13287-015-0150-x

7. Edelstein C, Pfaffinger D, Scanu AM (1984) Advantages and limitations of density gradient ultracentrifugation in the fractionation of human serum lipoproteins: role of salts and sucrose. J Lipid Res 25(6):630–637

8. Zhou H, Xu W, Qian H, Yin Q, Zhu W, Yan Y (2008) Circulating RNA as a novel tumor marker: an in vitro study of the origins and characteristics of extracellular RNA. Cancer Lett 259(1):50–60

9. Malik ZA, Kott KS, Poe AJ, Kuo T, Chen L, Ferrara KW et al (2013) Cardiac myocyte exosomes: stability, HSP60, and proteomics. Am J Phys Heart Circ Phys 304(7):H954–HH65

10. Balaj L, Atai NA, Chen W, Mu D, Tannous BA, Breakefield XO et al (2015) Heparin affinity purification of extracellular vesicles. Sci Rep 5:10266. https://doi.org/10.1038/srep10266

11. Wei ZY, Batagov AO, Carter DRF, Krichevsky AM (2016) Fetal bovine serum RNA interferes with the cell culture derived extracellular RNA. Sci Rep 6:31175. https://doi.org/10.1038/srep31175

12. Laurent LC, Abdel-Mageed AB, Adelson PD, Arango J, Balaj L, Breakefield X et al (2015) Meeting report: discussions and preliminary findings on extracellular RNA measurement methods from laboratories in the NIH Extracellular RNA Communication Consortium. J Extracell Vesicles 4:26533. https://doi.org/10.3402/jev.v4.26533

13. Yanez-Mo M, Siljander PR, Andreu Z, Zavec AB, Borras FE, Buzas EI et al (2015) Biological properties of extracellular vesicles and their physiological functions. J Extracell Vesicles 4:27066

14. Simonson B, Das S (2015) MicroRNA therapeutics: the next magic bullet? Mini Rev Med Chem 15(6):467–474

Chapter 4

Use of a Hollow Fiber Bioreactor to Collect Extracellular Vesicles from Cells in Culture

Irene K. Yan, Neha Shukla, David A. Borrelli, and Tushar Patel

Abstract

Current approaches for collection of extracellular vesicles (EV) are based on classical cell culture media production. This involves collection from cells grown in flasks, and can require multiple rounds of centrifugation or filtration, followed by ultracentrifugation or density gradient centrifugation. There are several limitations of these approaches, for example, they require a large input volume, the yield and concentration is low, and the process is time consuming. Most cell cultures require the use of fetal bovine serum which contains a large amount of endogenous EV that can contaminate isolations of cell-derived EVs. The use of cell cultures within a hollow fiber bioreactor could address many of these limitations and produce a continuous source of highly concentrated EVs without contamination from serum EVs, and that are suitable for downstream applications.

Key words Extracellular vesicles, Isolation, Hollow fiber bioreactor, Exosomes

1   Introduction

Many of the current approaches that are used for collection of extracellular vesicles (EV) are based on isolation from media obtained from classical cell culture approaches. This is commonly performed using cells grown in flasks, involves multiple rounds of centrifugation or filtration, followed by ultracentrifugation or velocity gradients. There are several limitations to these approaches, for example, they require a large input volume, the yield and concentration is low, and the process is time consuming. In addition to these limitations, one of the greatest challenges is the need to use fetal bovine serum (FBS) in cell culture media. Most cell cultures require the use of FBS, however, serum contains a large amount of endogenous EV, and these can contaminate isolations of EV released from cells that are cultured in media containing FBS.

Many of these limitations can be overcome with the use of a hollow fiber bioreactor. This is a three-dimensional culture system that comprises cells cultured within an enclosed system that can be

Tushar Patel (ed.), *Extracellular RNA: Methods and Protocols*, Methods in Molecular Biology, vol. 1740, https://doi.org/10.1007/978-1-4939-7652-2_4, © Springer Science+Business Media, LLC 2018

used for cell expansion in place of growth in flasks [1, 2]. The hollow fibers are small, semipermeable polysulfone membranes with a molecular weight cutoff that are bundled together in a tubular cartridge. The closed system has two compartments, an intracapillary space within the lumen of the fibers and an extracapillary space (ECS) surrounding the hollow fibers. These cartridges are loaded with cells into the ECS. Cells adhere to the outside of the hollow fibers and feed on the nutrients through perfusion within the intracapillary space. The hollow fibers provide a large surface area for cells to adhere, and the culture media is continuously pumped inside the fibers to allow for exchange of nutrients, gas, and waste (Fig. 1). Cells can be maintained in the system over long periods of time without the need to passage. Supernatant can be collected from the ECS and can be used for the isolation of EVs that are released from cells grown within the bioreactor. Most importantly, the use of serum-free media within the ECS could avoid contamination from EV within FBS. Adaptation of cells for growth in defined media without serum is necessary for this.

The use of hollow fiber bioreactor technology can produce a continuous source of highly concentrated EV from cells in culture [3, 4]. The process can be scaled up for further production or adapted for GMP compliant expansion [5].

2   Materials

1. Cells. Obtain cells and media to be used for cell culture (*see* **Note 1**). Cells can be adherent or grown in suspension cultures.

2. Cell culture media.

    (a) Basal medium (with no additives).

    (b) Complete medium (containing FBS, antibiotics, growth factors).

    (c) Serum-free medium.

3. Hollow fiber bioreactor.

    (a) Medium reservoir bottle.

    (b) Reservoir cap (*see* **Note 2**).

    (c) Perfusion pump.

    (d) Hollow fiber cartridge, e.g., 20 kDa Polysulfone Cartridge, FiberCell Systems.

4. Cell culture incubator at 37 °C.

5. Glucose measurements.

    (a) Glucose meter.

    (b) Glucose test strips.

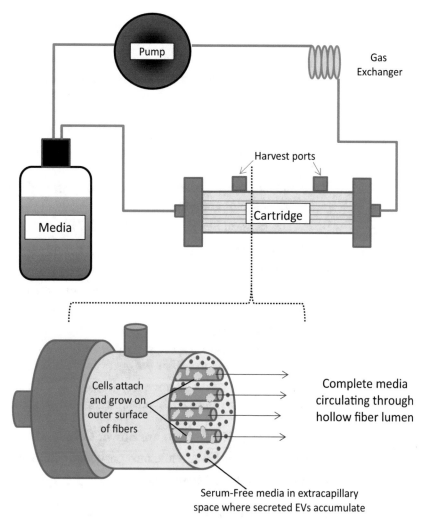

Fig. 1 Schematic diagram of hollow fiber bioreactor. The reservoir bottle contains medium. A perfusion pump circulates medium through the closed circuit. Fresh medium perfuses through the hollow fibers to nurture the cells growing within the cartridges. Cell growth can be monitored by metabolic products such as glucose and lactate that permeate into the circulating medium by gradient diffusion

6. Ultracentrifugation.
   (a) Beckman Coulter Optima™ L-80XP Ultracentrifuge.
   (b) Type 70Ti Rotor.
   (c) Polycarbonate ultracentrifuge tubes.
7. Other supplies.
   (a) 0.22 μm PES vacuum filter.
   (b) PBS.
   (c) 10–30 ml sterile disposable syringes.
   (d) Large bore needles.

3   Methods

3.1   Preparation of Hollow Fiber Culture System

1. Assemble the culture system as shown in Fig. 2 (*see* **Note 3**). First assemble the reservoir bottle and connect inlet and outlet tubing of hollow fiber cartridge to luer fittings on reservoir cap.

2. Insert reservoir cap into bottle of PBS. Make sure end port clamps are open and extracapillary space (ECS) side ports are closed.

3. Manually pump the compression tubing until circuit is filled and all bubbles are purged.

4. Fill the extracapillary space (ECS) with PBS.

5. Close end port clamps.

6. Fill 30 ml syringe with 30 ml PBS.

7. Attach syringe to one ECS side port and attach an empty syringe to other ECS side port.

8. Open both ECS ports.

9. Inject PBS from one syringe until cartridge is filled and some PBS is displaced into other syringe.

10. Detach syringes and remove any remaining PBS or displaced air. Reattach syringes back onto ports to use as caps.

3.2   Set Perfusion Flow Rate

1. Make sure ECS side ports are closed. Open end ports.

2. Assemble cartridge module into perfusion pump in incubator.

3. Turn flow rate to 20 ml/min.

3.3   Addition of Culture Media

1. Perfuse with PBS for at least 24 h.

2. Replace PBS with Basal Medium in reservoir and ECS for 24 h.

3. Replace Basal Medium with Complete Medium in reservoir.

4. Replace ECS with serum-free medium.

3.4   Cell Inoculation

1. Split and count cells. You will need $5-10 \times 10^7$ to inject into a C2011 cartridge (*see* **Note 4**). Use cells that are 90% viable and growing in a log phase. Prepare cells in 20 ml of serum-free media, and fill into a 20 ml syringe.

2. Close the left and right side ports of cartridge.

3. Remove both syringes.

4. Replace with one fresh 20 ml syringe and attach the syringe containing cells to the other port, and inject cells. Gently flush cell suspension back and forth between syringes.

5. Close one ECS port slide clamp and open one end port clamp and displace remaining media from syringes into reservoir.

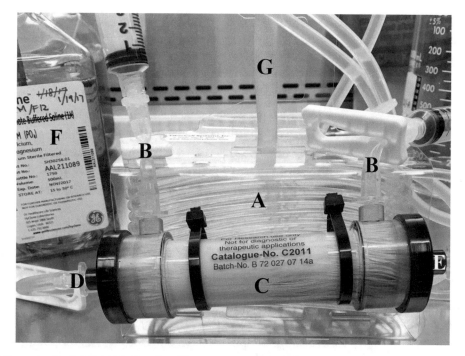

Fig. 2 Components of a typical hollow fiber bioreactor setup. The entire setup, including the perfusion pump, is within a temperature controlled cell culture incubator. (**a**) Gas exchange circulator; (**b**) Luer-Lok harvest and injection ports (shown with syringes attached); (**c**) Hollow fiber cartridge; (**d**) Circulating media inlet; (**e**) Circulating media outlet; (**f**) Complete media reservoir; (**g**) Tubing interface to perfusion pump (pump not shown)

6. Detach syringes and remove any remaining media or displaced air. Reattach syringes back onto ports to use as caps.

7. Replace reservoir with 125 ml of complete media, be sure to measure and record initial glucose level of media (*see* **Note 5**).

8. Make sure ECS port slide clamps are closed and end port slide clamps are open. Return system back to incubator and pump at 20 ml/min.

3.5 Bioreactor Maintenance

1. After cell inoculation, measure glucose level of reservoir bottle daily.

2. When glucose is depleted by 50%, replace with 250 ml of complete media.

3. Measure glucose daily, once this is depleted by half, replace with 500 ml of complete media and change pump speed to 30 ml/min.

4. Again, once the glucose is depleted by half, replace with 1 L of media (*see* **Note 6**).

5. Once glucose consumption is at 1 g/day, cells and supernatant may be harvested.

3.6 Harvest Cell Supernatant

1. Measure glucose consumption in samples from reservoir bottle to assess metabolic state and monitor cell growth (*see* **Note 5**). Supernatant can be harvested once glucose uptake is confirmed (*see* **Note 7**).

2. Fill a 10 ml syringe with fresh serum-free media.

3. Close ECS ports, and attach a fresh syringe to one port. Attach the syringe with fresh media to the other port.

4. Slowly displace serum-free media into the cartridge, while filling the empty syringe with supernatant from ESC.

5. Close clamps and transfer EV supernatant to 15 ml conical tube.

6. Spin supernatant at $300 \times g$ for 5 min.

7. Filter supernatant using a 0.22 µM syringe filter.

8. Process supernatant for EV isolation immediately (*see* **Note 8**), or store at 4 °C for up to 3 days.

3.7 Isolation of EV by Ultracentrifugation

1. Transfer 10 ml of supernatant to ultracentrifuge tube and fill up to 20 ml with PBS.

2. Centrifuge sample at $100,000 \times g$ for 70 min at 4 °C (*see* **Note 9**).

3. Remove supernatant and wash pellet with 20 ml PBS.

4. Centrifuge sample at $100,000 \times g$ for 70 min at 4 °C (*see* **Note 9**).

5. Remove supernatant and resuspend EV pellet in 100 µl PBS.

6. Store EV at −20 °C (*see* **Note 10**).

4 Notes

1. The optimal confluency and growth media needed for each cell type will need to be assessed separately for each different cell type. Adaptation of cells to basal defined media may be necessary prior to use of the hollow fiber culture system, with assessment of cell growth, morphology, viability, or other phenotypic features.

2. Reservoir cap is available in different sizes. Be sure to prepare the correct size depending on bottle neck.

3. Make sure all items are sterile and autoclaved. The life of the hollow fiber bioreactor system will be extended with the use of appropriate sterile technique to reduce contamination. All materials should be prepared in an aseptic setting.

4. The use of the hollow fiber cartridges will need to be optimized for each cell type. Polysulfone fibers are suitable for adherent or suspension cell lines. A 20 kDa MWCO can be used to concentrate extracellular vesicles and proteins greater than 120 kDa. There are two sizes of the 20 kDa cartridge available commercially, and the size used would depend on desired scale and cell number.

5. Unlike cells cultured in flasks, monitoring cell growth in hollow fiber bioreactors requires indirect assessments such as glucose consumption or lactate production [6, 7]. The rate of glucose consumption is related to the growth rate. Depletion can take up to several days, but if there is a slow consumption, cells may be in a static or quiescent stage.

6. Glucose levels can be measured using a glucometer and test strips.

7. EV can be isolated using any conventional approach used for isolation of EV from supernatant obtained from cells cultured in flasks [8–10].

8. EV RNA can be isolated using approaches described in chapter 3 by Bakr et al.

9. Retrieve sample from ultracentrifuge immediately after spin is complete.

10. EV sample should be used fresh for best results. Storage conditions may need to be optimized for long-term storage.

References

1. Gramer MJ, Poeschl DM (2000) Comparison of cell growth in T-flasks, in micro hollow fiber bioreactors, and in an industrial scale hollow fiber bioreactor system. Cytotechnology 34(1–2):111–119. https://doi.org/10.1023/A:1008167713696

2. Storm MP, Sorrell I, Shipley R, Regan S, Luetchford KA, Sathish J, Webb S, Ellis MJ (2016) Hollow fiber bioreactors for in vivo-like mammalian tissue culture. J Vis Exp (111). https://doi.org/10.3791/53431

3. Watson DC, Bayik D, Srivatsan A, Bergamaschi C, Valentin A, Niu G, Bear J, Monninger M, Sun M, Morales-Kastresana A, Jones JC, Felber BK, Chen X, Gursel I, Pavlakis GN (2016) Efficient production and enhanced tumor delivery of engineered extracellular vesicles. Biomaterials 105:195–205. https://doi.org/10.1016/j.biomaterials.2016.07.003

4. Tapia F, Vazquez-Ramirez D, Genzel Y, Reichl U (2016) Bioreactors for high cell density and continuous multi-stage cultivations: options for process intensification in cell culture-based viral vaccine production. Appl Microbiol Biotechnol 100(5):2121–2132. https://doi.org/10.1007/s00253-015-7267-9

5. Barckhausen C, Rice B, Baila S, Sensebe L, Schrezenmeier H, Nold P, Hackstein H, Rojewski MT (2016) GMP-compliant expansion of clinical-grade human mesenchymal stromal/stem cells using a closed hollow fiber bioreactor. Methods Mol Biol 1416:389–412. https://doi.org/10.1007/978-1-4939-3584-0_23

6. Curcio E, Piscioneri A, Salerno S, Tasselli F, Morelli S, Drioli E, Bartolo LD (2012) Human lymphocytes cultured in 3-D bioreactors: influence of configuration on metabolite transport and reactions. Biomaterials 33(33):8296–8303. https://doi.org/10.1016/j.biomaterials.2012.07.065

7. De Bartolo L, Salerno S, Curcio E, Piscioneri A, Rende M, Morelli S, Tasselli F, Bader A, Drioli E (2009) Human hepatocyte functions in a crossed hollow fiber membrane bioreactor. Biomaterials 30(13):2531–2543. https://doi.org/10.1016/j.biomaterials.2009.01.011

8. Kogure T, Lin WL, Yan IK, Braconi C, Patel T (2011) Intercellular nanovesicle-mediated microRNA transfer: a mechanism of environmental modulation of hepatocellular cancer cell growth. Hepatology 54(4):1237–1248. https://doi.org/10.1002/hep.24504

9. Kogure T, Patel T (2013) Isolation of extracellular nanovesicle microRNA from liver cancer cells in culture. Methods Mol Biol 1024:11–18. https://doi.org/10.1007/978-1-62703-453-1_2

10. Xu R, Simpson RJ, Greening DW (2017) A protocol for isolation and proteomic characterization of distinct extracellular vesicle subtypes by sequential centrifugal ultrafiltration. Methods Mol Biol 1545:91–116. https://doi.org/10.1007/978-1-4939-6728-5_7

Chapter 5

Isolation of Extracellular RNA from Serum/Plasma

Justyna Filant, Parham Nejad, Anu Paul, Bridget Simonson, Srimeenakshi Srinivasan, Xuan Zhang, Leonora Balaj, Saumya Das, Roopali Gandhi, Louise C. Laurent, and Anil K. Sood

Abstract

Extracellular RNAs are initiating increased interest due to their potentials in serving as novel biomarkers, mediators of intercellular communication, and therapeutic applications. As a newly emerging field, one of the main obstacles is the lack of standardized protocols for RNA isolations. Here we describe protocols for commercially available kits that have been modified to yield consistent results for isolation of extracellular RNA from both whole serum/plasma and extracellular vesicle-enriched serum/plasma samples.

Key words Cell biology, Extracellular RNA, Extracellular Vesicle, Nucleic acids, Molecular Biology, Isolation, Purification and separation

1 Introduction

Extracellular nucleic acids were first identified in human biofluids in 1948 [1]. Extracellular RNAs (exRNAs) play an important role in intercellular communication in the body. Various reports suggest that RNAs released from one tissue can alter expression in other cells [2]. Most of these exRNAs are noncoding RNAs of various types, many of which have no known function. These types of exRNAs include microRNAs (miRNAs), small interfering RNA (siRNA), piwi-interacting RNA (piRNA), long noncoding RNA (lncRNA), messenger RNA (mRNA) fragments, and transfer RNA (tRNA). It is widely thought that although "free" exRNA can be released from cells without associated macromolecules or a plasma membrane envelope, the ribonucleases present in the extracellular space would rapidly degrade free RNAs. Evidence of exRNA in biofluids suggests that they are protected from the environment through association

Justyna Filant, Parham Nejad, Anu Paul, Bridget Simonson, Srimeenakshi Srinivasan, Xuan Zhang, Leonora Balaj are Lab members (listed in alphabetical order).
Saumya Das, Roopali Gandhi, Louise C. Laurent, Anil K. Sood are Lab PI's (listed in alphabetical order).

Tushar Patel (ed.), *Extracellular RNA: Methods and Protocols*, Methods in Molecular Biology, vol. 1740,
https://doi.org/10.1007/978-1-4939-7652-2_5, © Springer Science+Business Media, LLC 2018

with extracellular vesicles such as exosomes, apoptotic bodies, microvesicles, lipoproteins, and ribonucleoproteins [3].

This chapter describes various RNA isolation methods that can be used to extract RNA from serum and/or plasma. exRNA association with extracellular particles necessitates specific techniques to enrich for each compartment. exRNA can be extracted either from whole serum/plasma or from vesicle-enriched serum/plasma. Vesicle enrichment can be done using one of the four methods, namely: precipitation, membrane filtration, affinity purification, and differential centrifugation.

Precipitation of extracellular vesicles can be done using the ExoQuick (System Biosciences) kit, which is based on the polyethylene glycol (PEG)/sodium chloride (NaCl) method for precipitating macromolecules. This method can precipitate extracellular vesicles as well as lipoprotein and ribonucleoprotein complexes [4]. Amicon ultracentrifugal filters (Millipore) can also be used to enrich for extracellular particles. These are based on size exclusion and hence will enrich all types of extracellular particles smaller than the pore size. This technique can be used to exclude larger particles such as microvesicles or apoptotic bodies. ExoRNeasy kit (Qiagen) uses membrane affinity spin columns for binding all types of extracellular vesicles [5]. New England Peptide's Vn96 peptide binds to heat-shock proteins on the exterior surface of exosomes and other extracellular vesicles and precipitates them through a series of centrifugation steps. Finally, ultracentrifugation can be used to enrich for extracellular vesicles by virtue of their density.

Following this, exRNA can be isolated either from the enriched biofluid or the total biofluid using multiple methods. Some of the methods described in this chapter are miRNeasy micro kit (Qiagen), Circulating RNA isolation kit (Norgen Biotek), miRCURY RNA isolation kit (Exiqon), and SeraMir exosome RNA purification kit (System Biosciences).

2 Materials

2.1 ExoQuick

1. ExoQuick Plasma Prep and Exosome Precipitation kit (System Biosciences EXOQ5TM-1).
2. Phosphate-buffered saline (PBS).

2.2 miRcury Exosome Plus

1. miRcury Biofluids kit (Exiqon—300112/300113).
2. miRcuryTM Exosome Isolation Kit—Serum and plasma (Exiqon—300101).
3. RNase-free water (Ambion—AM9937).

2.3 Millipore

Prepare all solutions using RNase-free water.

1. Qiagen miRNeasy micro kit (217084): Buffers RWT and RPE are supplied as concentrates. Before using for the first time, add the required volumes of 100% ethanol, as indicated on the bottle to obtain a working solution.

2. Chloroform.

3. 200 proof ethanol: 100% solution and freshly prepared 70% solution in water.

4. Phosphate-buffered saline (PBS).

5. AU-0.5 filter, 0.5 mL, 10 kDa MWCO (EMD Millipore—UFC501024).

2.4 ExoRNeasy

Prepare all solutions using RNase-free water.

1. ExoRNeasy Midi kit (Qiagen, 77044): Buffers RWT and RPE are supplied as concentrates. Before using for the first time, add the required volumes of 100% ethanol, as indicated on the bottle to obtain a working solution.

2. RNeasy MinElute Columns (Qiagen, Part of miRNeasy micro kit—217084).

3. Chloroform.

4. 200 proof ethanol: 100% solution and freshly prepared 70% solution in water.

2.5 ME Kit

1. New England Peptide ME™ kit—ME-010-kit.

2. Phosphate-buffered saline (PBS), pH 7.4.

3. Protease Inhibitor Cocktail, Set III EDTA-free (EMD)—539134.

4. Qiagen miRNeasy Micro kit—217084.

5. Chloroform (Sigma-Aldrich, 319988).

6. 100% ethanol (Koptec, V1016).

7. 70% ethanol.

8. RNase-free water (Ambion —AM9937).

2.6 Ultracentrifugation

1. Ultracentrifuge.

2. Swinging bucket rotor (TLA110/MLA5).

3. Qiagen miRNeasy micro kit (217084).

4. Chloroform (Sigma-Aldrich—319988).

5. 100% ethanol (Koptec—V1016).

6. 70% ethanol.

7. RNase-free water (Ambion—AM9937).

8. Phosphate Buffer Solution (PBS).

2.7 miRNeasy Micro Kit	1. Qiagen miRNeasy Micro kit (217084): Buffers RWT and RPE are supplied as concentrates. Before using for the first time, add the required volumes of 100% ethanol, as indicated on the bottle, to obtain the working solutions.

2. Chloroform.

3. 200 proof ethanol: 100% solution and freshly prepared 70% solution in water.

2.8 Norgen

1. Plasma/Serum Circulating and Exosomal RNA Purification Mini Kit (Norgen BioTek—51000).

2. 2-Mercaptoethanol, 99% Extra Pure (Acros Organics—125472500).

3. 100% ethanol (Koptec—V1016).

4. RNase-free water (Ambion—AM9937).

5. Optional: Amicon Ultra 0.5 mL Centrifugal filter devices—3K (Amicon—UFC500396).

2.9 miRcury Biofluids Kit

1. miRcury Biofluids kit (Exiqon—300112/300113)

2. Isopropanol (Sigma-Aldrich—I9516).

3. 100% ethanol (Koptec—V1016).

4. RNase-free water (Ambion—AM9937).

2.10 SeraMir

1. SeraMir Exosome RNA Purification Column Kit (System Biosciences—RA808A-1).

2. 100% ethanol (Koptec—V1016).

3. RNase-free water (Ambion—AM9937).

2.11 Equipment

1. Microfuge for centrifugation at 4 °C and at room temperature.

2. 1.5 mL Microfuge tubes.

3. 15 mL Centrifuge tubes.

4. Vortexer.

5. Phase lock gel tubes, 2 mL (VWR—10847-802).

3 Methods

3.1 ExoQuick

1. Transfer 500 μL of serum/plasma into a 1.5 mL microfuge tube.

   (a) For plasma, add 5 μL thrombin (500 U/mL) to a final concentration of 5 U/mL.

   (b) Incubate at room temperature for 5 min while mixing (gently flicking tube).

   (c) Centrifuge at $10,000 \times g$ for 5 min. There should be a visible fibrin pellet at the bottom of the tube.

   (d) Transfer supernatant to new microfuge tube.

2. Add 125 µL of ExoQuick Exosome Precipitation Solution to the serum and incubate for 30 min at 4 °C.

3. Centrifuge ExoQuick mixture at $1500 \times g$ for 30 min at room temperature.

4. Aspirate supernatant.

5. Spin down residual ExoQuick solution by centrifugation at $1500 \times g$ for 5 min at room temperature.

6. Remove all traces of fluid by aspiration, taking great care not to disturb the pellet.

7. Resuspend the pellet in 50 µL sterile PBS and proceed with RNA isolation using SeraMir Exosome RNA Purification Column Kit.

3.2 miRCURY Exosome Plus Kit

1. Add 200 µL of Precipitation Buffer A and vortex for 5 s.

2. Incubate for 60 min at 4 °C.

3. Spin for 30 min at $1500 \times g$ at room temperature.

4. Remove supernatant and discard (or save for comparative analysis).

5. Resuspend the pellet by vortexing in 270 µL of Resuspension Buffer ending up with ~300 µL of volume and proceed with the miRCURY™ RNA isolation kit—Biofluids

6. Mix 300 µL of resuspended exosomes with 90 µL of Lysis Buffer solution BF.

7. Vortex for 5 s.

8. Incubate for 10 min at room temperature.

9. Add 30 µL of Protein Precipitation Solution BF.

10. Vortex for 5 s.

11. Incubate for 1 min at room temperature.

12. Centrifuge for 3 min at $11,000 \times g$.

13. Transfer the clear supernatant into a new collection tube (2 mL, with lid).

14. Add 400 µL of isopropanol.

15. Vortex for 5 s.

16. Assemble the microRNA Spin Column BF and load sample onto column.

17. Incubate 2 min at room temperature.

18. Spin for 30 s at $11,000 \times g$. Discard flow-through.

19. Add 100 µL Wash Solution 1 BF.

20. Spin for 30 s at $11,000 \times g$. Discard flow-through.

21. Add 700 μL Wash Solution 2 BF.

22. Spin for 30 s at $11,000 \times g$. Discard flow-through.

23. Add 250 μl Wash Solution 2 BF.

24. Spin for 2 min at $11,000 \times g$. Transfer spin column to fresh microfuge tube.

25. Add 30 μL water directly onto the membrane of the spin column.

26. Incubate for 1 min at room temperature.

27. Spin for 1 min at $100 \times g$ followed by 1 min at $11,000 \times g$.

3.3 Millipore

Carry out all procedures at room temperature unless otherwise specified.

3.3.1 Exosome Isolation

1. Add 500 μL PBS to the AU-0.5 filter, cap, and centrifuge for 10 min at $14,000 \times g$.

2. Reverse the device and centrifuge for 2 min at $1000 \times g$ to remove the residual PBS from the filter.

3. Aspirate PBS from the collection tube.

4. Transfer 500 μL serum/plasma to the AU-0.5 filter and cap the device.

5. Centrifuge for 30 min at $14,000 \times g$. There should be ~15 μL sample remaining in the upper chamber.

6. Remove device from the centrifuge and empty the collection tube.

7. Add 0.5 mL PBS to the filter device and gently pipette sample multiple times to mix.

8. Centrifuge for 30 min at $14,000 \times g$.

9. Place filter upside down in a fresh microcentrifuge tube.

10. Centrifuge for 2 min at $2000 \times g$ (see **Note 1**) to transfer the sample to the collection tube. Discard filter.

3.3.2 RNA Isolation

Add 700 μL Qiazol sample in the collection tube and isolate RNA using the miRNeasy micro kit (starting from **step 3**).

3.4 ExoRNeasy

Carry out all procedures at room temperature unless otherwise specified.

3.4.1 Exosome Isolation

1. Transfer 500 μL of serum/plasma equilibrated to room temperature into a 1.5 mL microfuge tube.

2. Add 500 μL XBP and mix well immediately by gently inverting the tube five times.

3. Add 800 μL of sample/XBP mixture onto the exoEasy spin column and centrifuge for 1 min at 500 × *g*.

4. Repeat **step 3** until all mixture is added onto the column.

5. Discard flow-through.

6. Add 800 μL XWP to the exoEasy spin column.

7. Centrifuge for 5 min at 5000 × *g*. Discard the flow-through together with the collection tube.

8. Transfer the spin column to a fresh collection tube.

3.4.2   RNA Isolation

1. Add 700 μL Qiazol to the membrane of the spin column.

2. Centrifuge for 5 min at 5000 × *g*.

3. Transfer the flow-through, which is the lysate, to a PLG tube (*see* **Note 2**).

4. Vortex for 5 s.

5. Incubate at room temperature for 5 min.

6. Add 90 μL chloroform.

7. Shake vigorously for 15 s.

8. Incubate for 3 min at room temperature.

9. Centrifuge sample for 5 min at 12,000 × *g* at 4 °C.

10. Transfer the upper aqueous phase to a new microcentrifuge tube.

11. Carefully measure the aqueous phase and add 2 volumes of 100% ethanol.

12. Mix gently and thoroughly. Do not centrifuge and do not delay moving on to the next step.

13. Assemble a MinElute spin column in a new collection tube.

14. Load up to 700 μL of the mixture from **step 12**, including any precipitate that may have formed, onto the column.

15. Centrifuge for 15 s at 1000 × *g* (*see* **Note 3**) at room temperature (*see* **Note 4**).

16. Discard flow-through.

17. Repeat **steps 14–16** until entire sample has been loaded.

18. Make sure that ethanol has been added to RWT and RPE buffers.

19. Add 700 μL Buffer RWT to the RNeasy MinElute spin column.

20. Centrifuge for 15 s at ≥8000 × *g* at room temperature to wash the column.

21. Discard the flow-through.

22. Pipet 500 μL Buffer RPE onto the RNeasy MinElute spin column.

23. Centrifuge for 15 s at ≥8000 × g to wash the column.

24. Discard the flow-through.

25. Pipet 500 μL Buffer RPE onto the RNeasy MinElute spin column.

26. Centrifuge for 2 min at ≥8000 × g (≥10,000 rpm) at room temperature to wash the column.

27. Discard the collection tube with the flow-through (*see* **Note 5**).

28. Transfer the RNeasy MinElute spin column into a new 2 mL collection tube (supplied).

29. Open the lid of the spin column, and centrifuge at full speed (14,000 × g) for 5 min to dry the membrane (*see* **Note 6**).

30. Discard the collection tube with the flow-through.

31. Transfer the RNeasy MinElute spin column in a new 1.5 mL collection tube (supplied). Add 14–30 μL RNase-free water directly to the center of the spin column membrane (*see* **Note 7**).

32. Centrifuge for 1 min at full speed to elute the RNA (Optional: Centrifuge for 1 min at 100 × g followed by 1 min at full speed) (*see* **Note 8**).

3.5 ME

1. Reconstitute the Vn96 peptide to 2.5 μg/μL by adding 200 μL ME-buffer. Reconstitute the negative control Vn96-Scr peptide by adding 40 μL ME-buffer. Store at 4°°C.

2. Transfer 500 μL of serum/plasma into a 1.5 mL microfuge tube.

3. Add 500 μL PBS.

4. Mix thoroughly.

5. Add 5 μL protease inhibitor cocktail.

6. Centrifuge for 7 min at 10,000 × g at room temperature to remove debris.

7. Transfer supernatant to fresh tube, avoiding any pelleted material.

8. Add 20 μL reconstituted Vn96 peptide (use same amount of Vn96-Scr as a negative control).

9. Invert tube ten times.

10. Incubate at room temperature for 30 min on a rotator (*see* **Note 9**).

11. Centrifuge for 7 min at 10,000 × g at room temperature to pellet extracellular vesicles.

12. Carefully remove and discard supernatant.

13. Wash by adding 1 mL PBS + 5 μL protease inhibitor cocktail, inverting ten times, centrifuging for 7 min at 10,000 × g at

room temperature, and carefully removing and discarding supernatant.

14. Repeat **step 13**.

15. Resuspend pellet in 700 μL Qiazol and isolate RNA using miRNeasy micro kit.

3.6 Ultracentrifugation

3.6.1 Exosome Isolation

1. Start with 500 μL serum/plasma.

2. Bring up volume to fill ultracentrifuge tube (2.3–2.5 mL) with PBS.

3. Centrifuge for 70 min at 100,000 × g at 4 °C.

4. Discard supernatant, and resuspend pellet in PBS to fill ultracentrifuge tube.

5. Centrifuge for 70 min at 100,000 × g at 4 °C.

6. Discard supernatant.

7. Resuspend pellet in 50 μl PBS and store at −80 °C, or

8. Proceed to miRNeasy RNA isolation by adding 700 μL Qiazol to pellet.

3.7 miRNeasy Micro Kit

1. Transfer 500 μL of serum/plasma into a 15 mL centrifuge tube.

2. Add 2500 μL (5× volumes) of QIAzol Lysis Reagent (*see* **Note 10**).

3. Vortex 5 s.

4. *Optional:* Transfer to PLG tubes. You may need to divide a sample into several PLG tubes depending on the volume (*see* **Note 2**).

5. Incubate for 5 min at room temperature.

6. Add 500 μL chloroform.

7. Shake vigorously for 15 s.

8. Incubate for 3 min at room temperature.

9. Centrifuge sample for 15 min at 12,000 × g at **4 °C**.

10. Transfer the upper aqueous phase to a new 15 mL centrifuge tube (*see* **Note 11**). Avoid the white interphase.

11. Carefully measure the aqueous phase and add 1.5× volumes of 100% ethanol.

12. Mix gently and thoroughly. Do not centrifuge and do not delay moving on to the next step.

13. Assemble a MinElute spin column in a new collection tube.

14. Load up to 700 μL of the mixture from **step 12**, including any precipitate that may have formed, onto the column.

15. Spin for 15 s at 1000 × g (*see* **Note 3**) at room temperature (*see* **Note 4**).

16. Discard flow-through.

17. Repeat **steps 14–16** until entire sample has been loaded.

18. Make sure that ethanol has been added to RWT and RPE buffers as instructed in the manufacturer's manual.

19. Add 700 μL Buffer RWT to the RNeasy MinElute spin column.

20. Centrifuge for 15 s at 8000 × *g* at room temperature to wash the column.

21. Discard the flow-through.

22. Pipet 500 μL Buffer RPE onto the RNeasy MinElute spin column.

23. Centrifuge for 15 s at 8000 × *g* to wash the column.

24. Discard the flow-through.

25. Pipet 500 μL 80% ethanol (*see* **Note 12**) onto the RNeasy MinElute spin column.

26. Centrifuge for 2 min at ≥8000 × *g* (≥10,000 rpm) at room temperature to wash the column.

27. Discard the collection tube with the flow-through (*see* **Note 5**).

28. Transfer the RNeasy MinElute spin column into a new 2 mL collection tube (supplied).

29. Open the lid of the spin column, and centrifuge at full speed for 5 min to dry the membrane (*see* **Note 6**).

30. Discard the collection tube with the flow-through.

31. Transfer the RNeasy MinElute spin column into a new 1.5 mL collection tube (supplied).

32. Add 14 or 30 μL RNase-free water directly to the center of the spin column membrane (*see* **Note 7**).

33. Centrifuge for 1 min at full speed to elute the RNA. (Optional: Centrifuge for 1 min at 100 × *g* followed by 1 min at full speed.) (*see* **Note 8**).

3.8 Norgen

1. Set Incubator to 60 °C and warm PS Solution A, PS Solution B, and PS Solution C for 20 min to ensure no precipitates are present.

2. Add 50 mL of 96–100% ethanol to Wash Solution and check off box on bottle noting addition of ethanol.

3. Add 10 μL 2-Mercaptoethanol per 1 mL PS Solution B. (*see* **Note 13**).

4. Transfer 500 μL serum/plasma into a microfuge tube.

5. Add 100 μL PS Solution A (*see* **Note 14**) and 900 μL PS Solution B (containing 2-Mercaptoethanol).

6. Vortex for 15 s.

7. Incubate for 10 min at 60 °C.

8. Add 1.5 mL 100% Ethanol.

9. Vortex for 15 s.

10. Centrifuge for 30 s at 100 × g at room temperature. Carefully decant supernatant, discarding it. DO NOT disrupt pellet.

11. To the pellet add 750 μL PS Solution C.

12. Vortex for 15 s.

13. Incubate for 10 min at 60 °C.

14. Add 750 μL 100% Ethanol.

15. Vortex for 15 s.

16. Assemble a mini filter Spin Column with a collection tube.

17. Transfer 650 μL of the mixture to the Filter Column.

18. Centrifuge for 1 min at 16,000 × g at room temperature.

19. Discard flow-through.

20. Repeat **steps 17–19** until all of the mixture has been added to the Filter Column.

21. Add 400 μL Wash Solution to the column.

22. Centrifuge for 1 min at 16,000 × g at room temperature.

23. Discard flow-through.

24. Repeat **steps 21–23** two more times for a total of three washes.

25. Open the cap of the column and centrifuge for 3 min at 16,000 × g at room temperature to dry the column. Discard collection tube.

26. Transfer the spin column to a fresh 1.7 mL elution tube.

27. Apply 30 μL water to the column (*see* **Note 15**).

28. Centrifuge for 2 min at 300 × g at room temperature to load the solution onto the column.

29. Centrifuge for 3 min at 16,000 × g at room temperature to elute the RNA.

30. *Optional*: Cleanup by Amicon filtration

    (a) Dilute the eluted RNA with 320 μL DNA/RNA-free water.

    (b) Place the Amicon column into a collection tube. Load sample onto column.

    (c) Spin for 8 min at 14,000 × g at room temperature until the volume of the sample is ~20 μL.

    (d) Discard the flow-through.

    (e) Invert the column and place it into a new tube.

    (f) Centrifuge for 2 min at 8000 × g at room temperature.

    (g) The final volume should be ~20 μL. The sample can be further concentrated using a speed-vac.

3.9 miRCURY

1. Add 80 mL of 100% ethanol to "Wash Solution 2 BF."

2. Transfer 500 μL of serum/plasma into a 1.5 mL microfuge tube.

3. Add 150 μL "Lysis Solution BF."

4. Vortex for 5 s.

5. Incubate for 10 min at room temperature.

6. Add 50 μL of "Protein Precipitation Solution BF."

7. Vortex for 5 s.

8. Incubate for 1 min at room temperature.

9. Centrifuge sample for 5 min at 12,000 × g at room temperature.

10. Transfer the cleared supernatant to a new microcentrifuge tube, avoiding any precipitate.

11. Add 675 μL isopropanol.

12. Vortex for 5 s.

13. Assemble the microRNA Spin Column BF and load sample onto column.

14. Incubate 2 min at room temperature.

15. Spin for 30 s at 11,000 × g. Discard flow-through.

16. Add 100 μL Wash Solution 1 BF.

17. Spin for 30 s at 11,000 × g. Discard flow-through.

18. Add 700 μL Wash Solution 2 BF.

19. Spin for 30 s at 11,000 × g. Discard flow-through.

20. Add 250 μl Wash Solution 2 BF.

21. Spin for 2 min at 11,000 × g. Transfer spin column to fresh microfuge tube.

22. Add 30 μL water directly onto the membrane of the spin column.

23. Incubate for 1 min at room temperature.

24. Spin for 1 min at 100 × g followed by 1 min at 11,000 × g.

3.10 SeraMir

1. Add 350 μL Lysis Buffer to the resuspended exosome pellet and vortex 15 s.

2. Incubate for 5 min at room temperature.

3. Add 200 μL of 100% Ethanol.

4. Vortex 10 s.

5. Assemble spin column and collection tube. Transfer mixture to spin column.

6. Centrifuge for 1 min at 17,000 × g rpm at room temperature (check to see that the liquid has all flowed through; if not, spin longer).

7. Discard flow-through.

8. Repeat **steps 6** and **7** until all lysate has been spun.

9. Add 400 μL Wash Buffer.

10. Centrifuge for 1 min at 17,000 × *g* at room temperature (check to see that the liquid has all flowed through; if not, spin longer).

11. Discard flow-through.

12. Repeat **steps 9–11** once again (total of two washes).

13. Centrifuge for 2 min at 17,000 × *g* at room temperature to dry.

14. Transfer spin column to fresh microfuge tube.

15. Add 30 μL Elution Buffer or water directly to membrane in spin column.

16. Centrifuge for 2 min at 400 × *g* at room temperature (loads buffer onto membrane) (*see* **Note 8**).

17. Centrifuge for 1 min at 17,000 × *g* at room temperature to elute RNA.

4   Notes

1. The manufacturer's protocol suggests spinning at 1000 × *g*.

2. PLG makes separation of aqueous phase from the interface easier, and thus is particularly useful for large numbers of samples or less experienced personnel, but it is expensive.

3. The manufacturer's protocol is for 8000 × *g*, but some labs have found that 1000 × *g* for the binding step gives better results.

4. The centrifuge *must* be above 20 °C so that excessive precipitation does not occur.

5. After centrifugation, carefully remove the RNeasy MinElute spin column from the collection tube so that the column does not contact the flow-through. Otherwise, carryover of ethanol will occur and result in lower RNA yields.

6. To avoid damage to their lids, place the spin columns into the centrifuge with at least one empty position between columns. Orient the lids so that they point in a direction opposite to the rotation of the rotor (e.g., if the rotor rotates clockwise, orient the lids counterclockwise). It is important to dry the spin column membrane since residual ethanol may reduce RNA yields. Centrifugation with the lids open ensures that no ethanol is carried over during RNA elution.

7. As little as 10 μL RNase-free water can be used for elution if a higher RNA concentration is required, but the yield will be

reduced by approximately 20%. Do not elute with less than 10 μL RNase-free water, as the spin column membrane will not be sufficiently hydrated. The dead volume of the RNeasy MinElute spin column is 2 μL: elution with 14 μL RNase-free water results in a 12 μL eluate.

8. Centrifuging at a low speed first helps the solvent wet the surface of the membrane prior to the full-speed centrifuging step. This results in a better yield/RNA recovery from the membrane.

9. This is different from the manufacturer's protocol, which suggests 15 min at RT or overnight at 4 °C.

10. Adapted from miRNeasy serum kit—added 5× the volume of Qiazol.

11. If there is poor phase separation, the original biofluid can be diluted. To "rescue" the exRNA preparation, additional buffer, Qiazol, and chloroform can be added (maintaining the ratio 1:5:1).

12. 80% ethanol should be prepared with ethanol (96–100%) and RNase-free water.

13. If the kit will be used up within 3 months, the 2-Mercaptoethanol can be added directly to the Solution B bottle.

14. Solution A contains a resin and must be mixed well before addition to samples.

15. The manufacturer's protocol suggests eluting with 100 μL of Elution Solution A. This volume was selected to match that of other kits to enable fair comparisons. Eluting with larger volumes will lead to a better yield, but more dilute samples.

Acknowledgements

J.F. and A.S. were supported by NIH grant UH3 TR000943. P.N., A.P., and R.G. were supported by UH2-UH3 TR000890. B.S. and S.D. were supported by UH3TR000901. S.S. and L.L. were supported by U01 HL126494 and UH3 TR000906. X.Z. and L.B. were supported by U19 CA179463. Christina Bennett helped in proofreading and formatting the article.

References

1. Hoy AM, Buck AH (2012) Extracellular small RNAs: what, where, why? Biochem Soc Trans 40(4):886–890. https://doi.org/10.1042/BST20120019

2. Niu MC, Cordova CC, Niu LC, Radbill CL (1962) RNA-induced biosynthesis of specific enzymes. Proc Natl Acad Sci U S A 48(11):1964–1969

3. Vickers KC, Palmisano BT, Shoucri BM, Shamburek RD, Remaley AT (2011) MicroRNAs are transported in plasma and delivered to recipient cells by high-density lipoproteins. Nat Cell

Biol 13(4):423–433. https://doi.org/10.1038/ncb2210

4. Izzo C, Grillo F, Murador E (1981) Improved method for determination of high-density-lipoprotein cholesterol I. Isolation of high-density lipoproteins by use of polyethylene glycol 6000. Clin Chem 27(3):371–374

5. Enderle D, Spiel A, Coticchia CM, Berghoff E, Mueller R, Schlumpberger M, Sprenger-Haussels M, Shaffer JM, Lader E, Skog J, Noerholm M (2015) Characterization of RNA from exosomes and other extracellular vesicles isolated by a novel spin column-based method. PLoS One 10(8):e0136133. https://doi.org/10.1371/journal.pone.0136133

Chapter 6

Isolation of Extracellular RNA from Bile

Irene K. Yan, Valentin X. Berdah, and Tushar Patel

Abstract

The study of extracellular RNA has been recently reported as a tool for biomarker discovery. Extracellular vesicles can be isolated from different types of body fluids which contain protein, mRNA, and noncoding RNA. Extracellular RNA isolated from bile could be a useful tool for analyzing biliary tract diseases or cancer. Herein, we describe protocols based on modifications of commercially available kits for the collection, processing, and isolation of extracellular RNA from bile.

Key words Extracellular Vesicles, Bile, Isolation, Extracellular RNA, Exosomes

1 Introduction

Bile is a unique body fluid that is produced by the liver, and stored within the gallbladder or released into the small intestine. Bile contains cholesterol, bile acids and bilirubin, released from hepatocytes within the liver. Extracellular vesicles released from cells within the liver or from the lining epithelia of the biliary ducts can be detected within bile [1]. Their isolation and characterization may provide opportunities for the improved diagnosis of diseases affecting the biliary tract [2–4]. In particular, the diagnosis of malignancy within the biliary tract is particularly difficult because currently available techniques are not always able to render an accurate diagnosis with certainty. Approaches such as biopsy or cytology are limited to the desmoplastic nature of tumor cells lining the bile duct. The analysis of tumor cell-derived extracellular vesicles offers opportunities for their use as potential biomarkers of bile duct cancer [5, 6]. The ability to isolate RNA from bile is necessary in order to characterize biliary extracellular vesicle RNA content for this purpose.

We describe several different approaches that can be used for the isolation of extracellular RNA from bile that is suitable for downstream applications such as polymerase chain reaction or RNA sequencing (Fig. 1). For analysis of RNA associated with extracellular vesicles, a method for the enrichment of vesicles such

Tushar Patel (ed.), *Extracellular RNA: Methods and Protocols*, Methods in Molecular Biology, vol. 1740,
https://doi.org/10.1007/978-1-4939-7652-2_6, © Springer Science+Business Media, LLC 2018

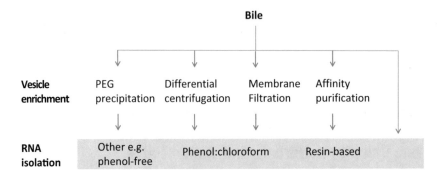

Fig. 1 Overview of approaches for the isolation of extracellular RNA or extracellular vesicle RNA from bile

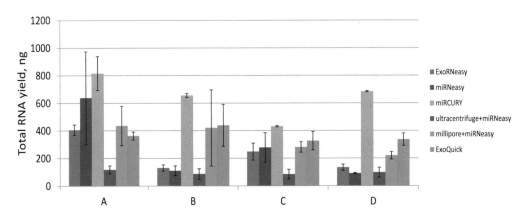

Fig. 2 Comparison of RNA yield using different exRNA isolation methods. Bile was obtained from patients with biliary tract cancer (**a, b**) or from patients without any biliary tract disease (**c, d**)

as the use of differential centrifugation, membrane filtration or affinity purification using spin columns, or precipitation using polyethylene glycolcan be performed first. RNA isolation from the vesicle-enriched portion, or from total bile can then be performed using phenol:chloroform or resin-based separations. Several kits are available for these. The yield of RNA obtained varies with the approach used (Fig. 2). The protocols described herein are modifications of these that have been useful for isolation of extracellular RNA or extracellular vesicle RNA from bile that is suitable for downstream applications such as PCR or RNA sequencing (Fig. 3).

2   Materials

2.1 Ultra-centrifugation

1. Ultracentrifuge (Beckman Coulter, XP-100).
2. Polyallomer ultracentrifuge tubes.
3. Swing bucket rotor, Type SW60Ti.
4. Phosphate buffered solution.

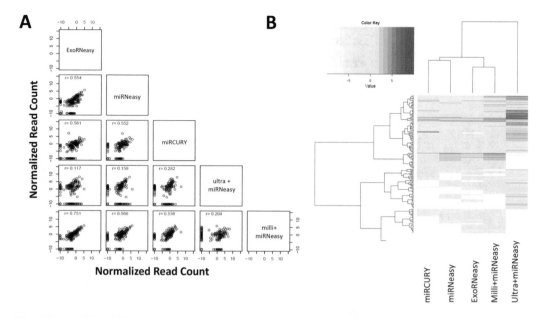

Fig. 3 Extracellular RNA was isolated from the bile of patient with a cholangiocarcinoma using each of five different isolation methods. RNA sequencing was performed and analysis performed using the normalized read counts of mature miRNA with ≥5 reads in all samples ($n = 186$). (**a**) Pearson correlation and (**b**) Heatmap of mapped mature miRNA reads from RNA sequencing obtained using each method are shown

2.2 Membrane Filtration

1. AU-05 filter, 0.5 ml, 10 kDa MWCO (Millipore).

2.3 Choice of RNA Isolation Kit

1. miRNeasy Micro Kit (Qiagen)—phenol:chloroform-based approach.

2. miRCURY RNA Isolation Kit—Biofluids (Exiqon)—resin-based separation.

3. ExoRNeasy MidiKit (Qiagen)—membrane affinity spin column-based separation.

4. SeraMir Exosome RNA Purification Kit (System Biosciences)—phenol-free RNA purification.

   (a) ExoQuick Precipitation Kit (System Biosciences)—PEG-based separation.

2.4 Other Reagents

1. Chloroform.

2. Absolute ethanol.

3 Methods

3.1 Collection and Storage of Bile

1. Bile can be collected into a sterile collection bottle by aspiration from a biliary catheter placed within the bile duct, or from

an external collection bag draining an indwelling biliary tube (*see* **Note 1**).

2. Centrifuge sample at $3000 \times g$ for 10 min at 4 °C to remove cellular sediment and debris.

3. Transfer supernatant into 1 ml aliquots in microcentrifuge tubes.

4. Store at 4 °C or −20 °C for long-term storage (>2 days).

5. RNA Isolation can be performed following ultracentrifugation, filtration, or directly using one of the other RNA isolation options (Subheadings 3.4–3.6) depending on specific application. Each of these approaches may potentially identify distinct RNA populations. Ultracentrifugation (Subheading 3.2) and use of Seramir and Exoquick (Subheading 3.7) may enrich for RNA within vesicles (extracellular vesicle RNA), where direct RNA isolation approaches (Subheadings 3.4–3.6) may isolate both vesicular and extra-vesicular RNA (extracellular RNA) (Fig. 1).

3.2 Ultra-centrifugation

1. Add 200 μl bile to ultracentrifuge tube (*see* **Note 2**).

2. Fill up to 4 ml with PBS.

3. Ultracentrifuge at $100,000 \times g$ for 70 min at 4 °C.

4. Remove supernatant and wash pellet with 1 ml PBS.

5. Add 3 ml of PBS, ultracentrifuge at $100,000 \times g$ for 70 min at 4 °C, and discard supernatant.

6. The pellet can be directly lyzed with 1000 μl QIAzol Lysis Reagent from miRNeasy kit.

7. Proceed with RNA isolation using miRNeasy kit method, Subheading 3.4, **step 3**.

3.3 Filtration

1. Add 500 μl PBS to the Millipore AU-0.5 filter and centrifuge at $14,000 \times g$ for 10 min at room temperature.

2. Discard flow-through, reverse filter, and centrifuge at $1000 \times g$ for 2 min to remove residual PBS from filter.

3. Combine 200 μl bile (*see* **Note 2**) and 300 μl PBS to the AU-0.5 filter and centrifuge at $14,000 \times g$ for 30 min at room temper-ature.

4. Add 500 μl PBS and spin for additional 30 min at $14,000 \times g$.

5. Transfer remaining sample from the filter (approximately 15 μl) to a new tube.

6. Add 1000 μl QIAzol Lysis Reagent, vortex 5 s, incubate for 5 min at room temperature.

7. Proceed with RNA isolation using miRNeasy kit method, Subheading 3.4, **step 2**.

3.4 miRNeasy Micro Kit

1. If starting with bile directly, transfer 200 µl of bile into 1.5 ml microcentrifuge tube (*see* **Note 2**).

2. Add 1000 µl QIAzol Lysis Reagent, vortex 5 s, incubate for 5 min at room temperature.

3. Add 200 µl chloroform, shake vigorously for 15 s and incubate for 3 min at room temperature.

4. Centrifuge sample at $12,000 \times g$ for 15 min at 4 °C.

5. Transfer the upper aqueous phase to a new microcentrifuge tube.

6. Add 500 µl 100% ethanol, mix by pipetting.

7. Assemble RNeasy Micro Column from kit in a new collection tube and load 700 µl of sample onto column.

8. Centrifuge sample at $8000 \times g$ for 15 s at room temperature (*see* **Note 3**). Discard flow-through and return column to collection tube.

9. Load remainder of sample onto column and repeat **step 8** of Subheading 3.4.

10. Add 700 µl Buffer RPE from kit to column and centrifuge at $8000 \times g$ for 15 s at room temperature. Discard flow-through and return column to collection tube.

11. Add 500 µl Buffer RPE from kit to column and centrifuge at $8000 \times g$ for 2 min at room temperature. Discard flow-through and return column to collection tube.

12. Centrifuge column at $8000 \times g$ for 1 min at room temperature to dry membrane (*see* **Note 4**).

13. Transfer spin column into a new collection tube.

14. Add 30 µl RNase-free H_2O from kit directly onto the membrane of spin column (*see* **Note 5**).

15. Close lid and centrifuge for 1 min at $8000 \times g$ at room temperature.

16. Discard spin column and store purified RNA at −70 °C.

3.5 miRCURY RNA Isolation

1. Transfer 200 µl of bile into 1.5 ml microcentrifuge tube (*see* **Note 2**).

2. Add 60 µl Lysis Solution from kit, vortex for 5 s and incubate for 3 min at room temperature.

3. Add 20 µl Protein Precipitation Solution from kit, vortex for 5 s, and incubate for 1 min at room temperature.

4. Centrifuge samples at $11,000 \times g$ for 3 min at room temperature (*see* **Note 3**).

5. Transfer clear supernatant to new microcentrifuge tube.

6. Add 270 µl Isopropanol and vortex for 5 s.

7. Assemble microRNA Mini Spin Column from kit in a new collection tube and load entire sample onto column.

8. Centrifuge at $11,000 \times g$ for 30 s at room temperature. Discard flow-through and return column to collection tube.

9. Add 700 μl Wash Solution 2 from kit to column and centrifuge at $11,000 \times g$ for 30 s at room temperature. Discard flow-through and return column to collection tube.

10. Add 250 μl Wash Solution 2 from kit to column and centrifuge at $11,000 \times g$ for 2 min at room temperature. Discard flow-through and return column to collection tube.

11. Add 50 μl rDNase from kit directly onto membrane of spin column.

12. Close lid and incubate for 15 min at room temperature.

13. Add 100 μl Wash Solution 1 from kit to column and centrifuge at $11,000 \times g$ for 30 s at room temperature. Discard flow-through and return column to collection tube.

14. Add 700 μl Wash Solution 2 from kit to column and centrifuge at $11,000 \times g$ for 30 s at room temperature. Discard flow-through and return column to collection tube.

15. Add 250 μl Wash Solution 2 from kit to column and centrifuge at $11,000 \times g$ for 2 min at room temperature (*see* **Note 4**).

16. Transfer spin column into a new microcentrifuge tube.

17. Add 50 μl RNase-free H_2O from kit directly onto the membrane of spin column (*see* **Note 5**).

18. Close lid and incubate for 1 min at room temperature.

19. Centrifuge at $11,000 \times g$ for 1 min at room temperature.

20. Discard spin column and store purified RNA at −70 °C.

3.6 ExoRNeasy MidiKit RNA Isolation

1. Transfer 200 μl of bile into 1.5 ml microcentrifuge tube (*see* **Note 2**).

2. Add 500 μl XBP from kit and mix well by inverting.

3. Transfer mixture into exoEasy spin column from kit and centrifuge at $500 \times g$ for 1 min.

4. Discard flow-through.

5. Add 800 μl XWP from kit to the exoEasy column and centrifuge at $5000 \times g$ for 5 min at room temperature.

6. Transfer exoEasy column to new collection tube.

7. Add 700 μl QIAzol Lysis Reagent from kit to the membrane of the exoEasy column.

8. Centrifuge at $5000 \times g$ for 5 min at room temperature.

9. Transfer flow-through to new tube, vortex 5 s, incubate for 5 min at room temperature.

10. Add 140 μl chloroform, shake vigorously for 15 s, incubate for 3 min at room temperature.

11. Centrifuge sample at 12,000 × *g* for 15 min at 4 °C.

12. Transfer the upper aqueous phase to a new microcentrifuge tube.

13. Add 500 μl 100% ethanol, mix by pipetting.

14. Assemble RNeasy Micro Column from kit in a new collection tube and load entire sample onto column.

15. Centrifuge sample at 8000 × *g* for 15 s at room temperature. Discard flow-through and return column to collection tube.

16. Add 700 μl Buffer RPE from kit to column and centrifuge at 8000 × *g* for 15 s at room temperature. Discard flow-through and return column to collection tube.

17. Add 500 μl Buffer RPE from kit to column and centrifuge at 8000 × *g* for 2 min at room temperature. Discard flow-through and return column to collection tube.

18. Centrifuge column at 8000 × *g* for 1 min at room temperature to dry membrane (*see* **Note 4**).

19. Transfer spin column into a new collection tube.

20. Add 30 μl RNase-free H$_2$O from kit directly onto the membrane of spin column (*see* **Note 5**).

21. Close lid and centrifuge for 1 min at 8000 × *g* at room temperature.

22. Discard spin column and store purified RNA at −70 °C.

3.7 SeraMir Exosome RNA Purification Kit

1. Transfer 200 μl of bile into 1.5 ml microcentrifuge tube (*see* **Note 2**).

2. Add 40 μl ExoQuick, mix well, incubate for 30 min at 4 °C.

3. Centrifuge sample at 16,000 × *g* for 2 min at 4 °C.

4. Remove supernatant, add 140 μl Lysis Buffer to pellet, vortex 15 s, incubate for 5 min at room temperature.

5. Add 80 μl 100% ethanol, vortex 10 s.

6. Assemble spin column from kit in a new collection tube and load entire sample onto column.

7. Centrifuge sample at 16,000 × *g* for 1 min at room temperature. Discard flow-through and return column to collection tube.

8. Add 400 μl Wash Buffer from kit to column and centrifuge at 16,000 × *g* for 1 min at room temperature. Discard flow-through and return column to collection tube. Repeat this entire step one more time.

9. Centrifuge column at $16,000 \times g$ for 2 min at room temperature to dry membrane (*see* **Note 3**).

10. Transfer spin column into a new collection tube.

11. Add 30 µl Elution Buffer from kit directly onto the membrane of spin column (*see* **Note 5**).

12. Close lid and centrifuge at $350 \times g$ for 2 min at room temperature.

13. Increase speed and centrifuge at $16,000 \times g$ for 1 min at room temperature.

14. Discard spin column and store purified RNA at $-70\ ^\circ$C.

4 Notes

1. Ensure that collection of bile is done using a sterile procedure to avoid contamination of bile with microorganisms.

2. The yield of RNA will depend on the input volume of bile used. A larger input volume of bile can be considered (up to 500 µl) based on application.

3. It is critical that centrifuge is set to room temperature to avoid precipitation.

4. Make sure columns are dry to avoid the carryover of ethanol.

5. To increase concentration of RNA, a lower amount of water can be used for elution. However, the total yield will be decreased.

Acknowledgments

This work was supported by the Office of the Director, National Institutes of Health (USA) through award UH3 TR000884. We acknowledge the expert assistance of Caitlyn Foerst and thank the members of our laboratories for their contributions.

Disclosures: None.

References

1. Maji S, Matsuda A, Yan IK, Parasramka M, Patel T (2017) Extracellular vesicles in liver diseases. Am J Physiol Gastrointest Liver Physiol 312(3):G194–G200. https://doi.org/10.1152/ajpgi.00216.2016

2. Gradilone SA, O'Hara SP, Masyuk TV, Pisarello MJ, LaRusso NF (2015) MicroRNAs and benign biliary tract diseases. Semin Liver Dis 35(1):26–35. https://doi.org/10.1055/s-0034-1397346

3. Marin JJ, Bujanda L, Banales JM (2014) MicroRNAs and cholestatic liver diseases. Curr Opin Gastroenterol 30(3):303–309. https://doi.org/10.1097/MOG.0000000000000051

4. Munoz-Garrido P, Garcia-Fernandez de Barrena M, Hijona E, Carracedo M, Marin JJ, Bujanda L, Banales JM (2012) MicroRNAs in biliary diseases. World J Gastroenterol 18(43):6189–6196. https://doi.org/10.3748/wjg.v18.i43.6189

5. Mayr C, Beyreis M, Wagner A, Pichler M, Neureiter D, Kiesslich T (2016) Deregulated MicroRNAs in biliary tract cancer: functional targets and potential biomarkers. Biomed Res Int 2016:4805270. https://doi.org/10.1155/2016/4805270

6. Haga H, Yan I, Takahashi K, Wood J, Patel T (2014) Emerging insights into the role of microRNAs in the pathogenesis of cholangiocarcinoma. Gene Expr 16(2):93–99. https://doi.org/10.3727/105221614X13919976902174

Chapter 7

Cushioned–Density Gradient Ultracentrifugation (C-DGUC): A Refined and High Performance Method for the Isolation, Characterization, and Use of Exosomes

Kang Li, David K. Wong, King Yeung Hong, and Robert L. Raffai

Abstract

Exosomes represent one class of extracellular vesicles that are thought to be shed by all cell types. Although the exact nature of exosome biogenesis and function remains incompletely understood, they are increasingly recognized as a source of intercellular communication in health and disease. Recent observations of RNA exchange via donor cell-derived exosomes that exert genetic regulation in recipient cells have led to a boon into exosome research. The excitement and promise of exosomes as a new therapeutic avenue for human pathologies remain limited by challenges associated with their isolation from culture media and biofluids. The introduction of new methodologies to facilitate the isolation of exosomes has simultaneously raised concerns related to the reproducibility of studies describing exosome effector functions. Even high-speed ultracentrifugation, the first and long considered gold standard approach for exosome isolation has recently been noted to be subject to uncontrolled variables that could impact functional readouts of exosome preparations. This chapter describes principles and methods that attempt to overcome such limitations by first concentrating exosomes in a liquid cushion and subsequently resolving them using density gradient ultracentrifugation. Our approach avoids possible complications associated with direct pelleting onto plastic tubes and allows for further purification of exosomes from dense protein aggregates.

Key words Exosomes, Density gradient ultracentrifugation, Flow cytometry, Nanoparticle tracking analysis, Iodixanol

1 Introduction

Exosomes are nano-sized membrane vesicles of endocytic origin that are secreted by almost all cell types and are abundantly present in body fluids [1]. The study of exosomes has recently attracted immense interest owing to their capacity to carry and transfer a variety of cell-signaling molecules including protein and RNA [2, 3]. Exosomes have thus become firmly recognized as vehicles for intercellular communication in health and in disease. Moreover, exosomes represent an ideal source of diagnostic biomarkers and a potential delivery vehicle for therapeutic applications [4, 5].

Tushar Patel (ed.), *Extracellular RNA: Methods and Protocols*, Methods in Molecular Biology, vol. 1740,
https://doi.org/10.1007/978-1-4939-7652-2_7, © Springer Science+Business Media, LLC 2018

A major challenge in this rapidly evolving field is the lack of a robust approach to isolate exosomes with high purity and biophysical integrity. Ever since the discovery of exosomes [6], ultracentrifugation has remained a commonly used approach to isolate these extracellular vesicles in a non-biased manner [7]. This procedure, however, does not discriminate between exosome subtypes and larger microvesicles, as well as from other nanoparticles, or even large protein aggregates [8–10]. Furthermore, the physical and biological integrity of exosomes isolated by ultracentrifugation may be compromised due to nanoparticle aggregation [8], high hydrostatic pressures caused by direct pelleting, and shear forces during dispensing [11]. As such, this method that has long been accepted as a gold standard for exosome isolation could be subject to substantial qualitative and quantitative variability. Such limitations could subsequently impact on downstream analyses, making it difficult to compare, reproduce, and interpret results of experiments performed across laboratories with exosomes prepared using this method [11]. As recently highlighted in a commentary by the EV-TRACK Consortium, there is a pressing need to develop methodologies to isolate and study the function of exosomes in a consistent and reproducible manner [12].

To address this issue, we built on numerous prior reports [13–16] and devised a robust methodological platform to isolate exosomes with high yield, purity, and integrity. We termed our method: Cushioned–Density Gradient Ultracentrifugation (C-DGUC). Our approach, illustrated in Figs. 1 and 2, offers multiple advantages over traditional ultracentrifugation of biofluids and culture media. First, the use of a 60% iodixanol cushion during the nanoparticle concentration step maximizes exosome recovery and allows for a better preservation of their physical integrity and biological activity by preventing pellet formation in the centrifuge tube. Second, the use of density gradient ultracentrifugation provides for high-quality exosome purification by efficiently removing non-exosome nanoparticles and protein contaminates (~90% of total protein, Fig. 3). Lastly, the biological inertness and compatibility of iodixanol with most downstream in vitro functional assays and even use in animals allow for reliable and efficient biochemical and physiological study of purified exosomes without the need for its removal. Fractions taken from iodixanol gradients can be readily analyzed for protein, nanoparticle, and RNA content by SDS-PAGE (Fig. 4a), western blotting (Fig. 4b), flow cytometry (Fig. 5), nanoparticle tracking analysis (Fig. 6), and microchip capillary electrophoresis (Fig. 7) all without a need for dialysis. The protocol detailed below represents a practical example of exosome isolation from mouse bone marrow-derived macrophage culture supernatants using our C-DGUC method. It is noteworthy that this method could be extended to exosome isolation from biofluids including plasma and urine for clinical research and diagnostic applications.

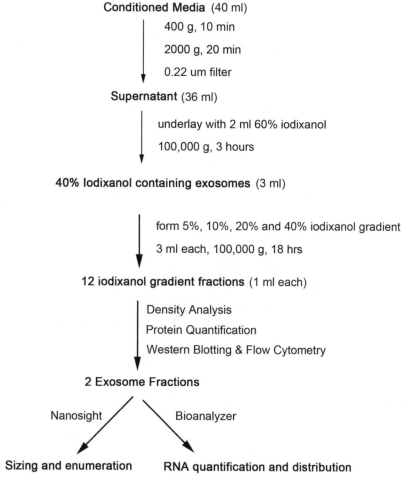

Fig. 1 Experimental workflow of cushioned–density gradient ultracentrifugation (C-DGUC) for exosome isolation

---

2 Materials

2.1 Macrophage Culture

1. Complete DMEM media: Dulbecco's modified Eagle's medium (DMEM) (Corning, 10-014), fetal bovine serum (Gibco), GlutaMax (Gibco), Penicillin-Streptomycin (Gibco).

2. Recombinant murine M-CSF (Peprotech).

3. Cell strainer, 70 μm (BD).

4. Non-treated cell culture dish (Corning).

5. D-PBS (Corning).

6. ACK lysing buffer (Lonza).

7. Cellstripper solution (Corning).

8. Exosome-free media (*see* **Note 1**).

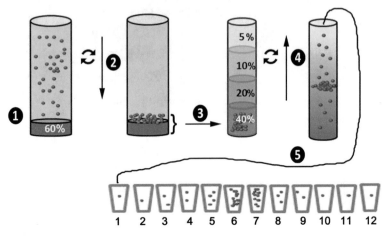

Fig. 2 Schematic illustration of C-DGUC for exosome isolation (*1*). Place a 2 mL solution of 60% iodixanol below the pre-cleared conditioned medium that serves to cushion the nanoparticles during centrifugation; (*2*) sediment the nanoparticles at 100,000 × *g* for 3 h; (*3*) remove the 2 mL cushion along with 1 mL of overlaying medium and place it below a pre-formed step density gradient composed of three layers of iodixanol solution, 3 mL each; (*4*) perform density gradient ultracentrifugation at 100,000 × *g* for a period of 18 h; (*5*) collect the medium from the top of the tube in 1 mL increments. Exosomes derived from cultured primary BMDM typically are isolated in fractions 6 and 7

2.2 Density Gradient Centrifugation

1. OptiPrep density gradient medium (60% iodixanol) (Sigma) (*see* **Note 2**).

2. Homogenization buffer: 0.25 M sucrose, 1 mM EDTA, 10 mM Tris–HCl, pH 7.4.

3. 50% Iodixanol (*see* **Note 3**).

4. Beckman floor-mode ultracentrifuge Optima XPN 90.

5. Beckman SW 28 Ti rotor.

6. Beckman SW 40 Ti rotor (*see* **Note 4**).

7. Beckman ultracentrifuge tubes.

8. 10 mL BD disposable syringe (BD).

9. 50 mL Steriflip-GP filter unit (Millipore).

10. Metal hub blunt point needles, 4-in. (Hamilton).

2.3 Fraction Analysis

1. Qubit protein assay Kit (Thermo Fisher Scientific).

2. Qubit 3.0 fluorometer (Thermo Fisher Scientific).

3. Nanosight LM14 (Malvern Instruments).

2.4 SDS-PAGE and Western Blotting

1. ImageQuant LAS 4000.

2. Anti-TSG101 antibody (Santa Cruz Biotechnology, sc-7964).

3. Anti-Alix antibody (Cell Signaling Technology, 2171).

4. IRDye 680RD goat anti-mouse IgG (LI-COR).

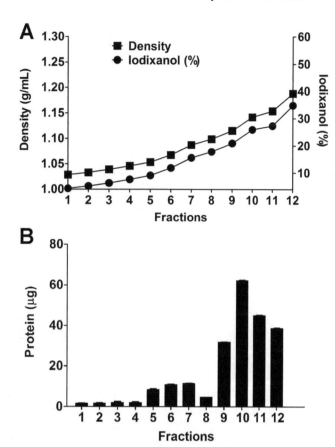

Fig. 3 Density analysis and protein quantitation of iodixanol gradient fractions. (**a**) The density and iodixanol percentage gradually increase in the 12 fractions collected from the top to the bottom of the gradient; (**b**) protein quantification in the 12 gradient fractions was performed by using Qubit Protein Assay

   5. IRDye 800CW goat anti-rabbit IgG (LI-COR).

   6. Odyssey infrared imaging system.

2.5 Flow Cytometry

   1. FITC anti-mouse CD81 antibody (Thermo Fisher Scientific, HMCD8101).

   2. Alexa Fluor 647 anti-mouse CD9 antibody (BioLegend, 124810).

   3. Sulfate latex beads, 4% w/v, 5 μm (Thermo Fisher Scientific).

   4. Glycine 1 M solution (Sigma).

   5. Bovine serum albumin (BSA), 7.5% w/v (Sigma).

2.6 Exosome RNA Analysis

   1. mirVana™ PARIS™ RNA and Native Protein Purification Kit (Thermo Fisher Scientific).

   2. Agilent 2100 bioanalyzer instrument.

   3. Agilent RNA 6000 pico kit.

   4. Agilent small RNA kit.

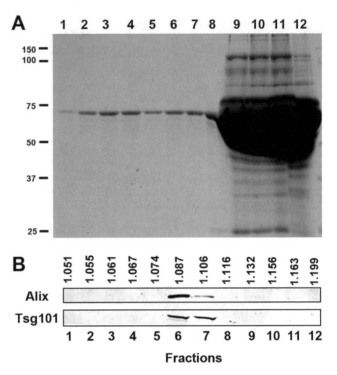

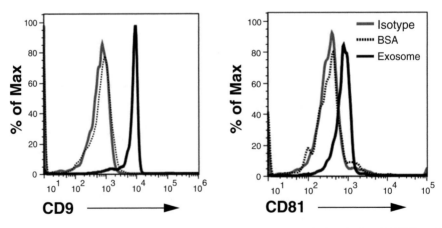

Fig. 4 Protein characterization of iodixanol gradient fractions. (**a**) SDS-PAGE analysis of gradient fractions. Fractions 1–12 (90 μL) were loaded. (**b**) Western blot analysis of gradient fractions for the exosome marker proteins Alix and Tsg101. Exosome proteins were observed in fractions 6–7

Fig. 5 Exosome characterization by flow cytometry. Exosomes (10 μg) were isolated by C-DGUC and nonspecifically captured on latex beads, immune-stained and analyzed by flow cytometry. Flow cytometry dot plots show positivity for exosomes markers CD9 and CD81

3   Methods

3.1 Preparation of Macrophage-Conditioned Media

1. Prepare single cell suspension from mouse bone marrow and pass cells through 70 μm cell strainer.

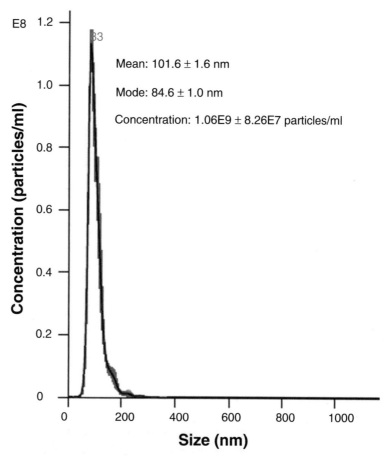

Mean: 101.6 ± 1.6 nm

Mode: 84.6 ± 1.0 nm

Concentration: 1.06E9 ± 8.26E7 particles/ml

Fig. 6 Exosome enumeration and sizing by nanoparticle tracking analysis. Exosomes-containing fractions 6 and 7 were pooled and diluted at 1:200 before analysis using the Nanosight LM14 instrument. A sharp peak at 84 nm was observed

2. Centrifuge at $300 \times g$ for 10 min at 4 °C and resuspend cells in 1 mL of ACK buffer to lyse red blood cells.

3. Incubate for 5 min at room temperature.

4. Add 10 mL D-PBS and centrifuge at $300 \times g$ for 10 min. Decant the supernatant and Add 25 mL complete DMEM media supplemented with M-CSF (40 ng/mL). Culture the cells in a 150-mm cell culture dish in a 37 °C incubator with 5% CO_2.

5. After 7 days of culture, decant the supernatant; add 3 mL Cellstripper to the cells.

6. Incubate for 5 min in 37 °C incubator. Gently tap the dishes to detach the cells.

7. Add 20 mL D-PBS, and transfer the cells to 50 mL tube and centrifuge at $300 \times g$ for 10 min. Decant the supernatant and resuspend the cells in 25 mL serum-free DMEM. Count the

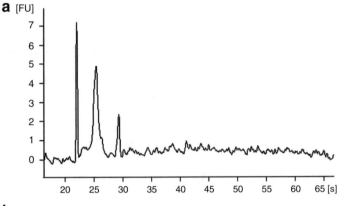

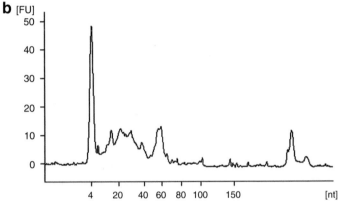

Fig. 7 Exosomal RNA characterization by Agilent bioanalyzer. Representative images of Agilent RNA 6000 Pico chip (**a**) and Small RNA chip (**b**) assays of total RNA isolated from macrophages-derived exosomes

cells and place 1.5×10^7 cells into a fresh 150-mm cell culture dish.

8. After 2 h, decant the supernatant and wash the cells three times with D-PBS, add 20 mL exosome-free media.

9. After 24–48 h, collect conditioned media into 50-mL conical tubes.

3.2 Nanoparticle Concentration on 60% Iodixanol Cushion

1. Combine the conditioned media from two 150-mm cell culture dishes and centrifuge the 40 mL media at $300 \times g$ for 10 min at 4 °C. Aspirate and transfer 38 mL media from the top to a fresh 50-mL conical tube; be careful NOT to disturb the pellet.

2. Centrifuge at $2000 \times g$ for 10 min at 4 °C to remove large cellular debris. Aspirate and transfer 36 mL media from the top to a fresh 50-mL conical tube; be careful NOT to disturb the pellet.

3. Filter the supernatant by passing through a 50 mL Steriflip-GP filter unit (0.22 μm) to remove remaining cell debris and large vesicles (*see* **Note 5**).

4. Add the 36 mL pre-cleared media into ultracentrifuge tube (*see* **Note 6**); carefully underlay the media with 2 mL of 60% iodixanol using Hamilton blunt point 4-in. needles (*see* **Note 7**).

5. After balancing the tubes within 0.1 g of each other, centrifuge in an SW 28 Ti rotor at $100,000 \times g$ for 2–4 h in Optima XPN 90 ultracentrifuge at 4 °C (*see* **Note 8**).

6. Carefully use blunt end needles to collect a volume of 3 mL from the bottom of the ultracentrifuge tubes that consists of 2 mL iodixanol cushion and 1 mL media, resulting in a mixture of 40% iodixanol. Mix thoroughly.

3.3 Exosome Isolation by Density Gradient Ultracentrifugation

1. Prepare 5%, 10%, and 20% iodixanol by mixing defined volumes of 50% Iodixanol with homogenization buffer according to Table 1, and allow 30 min mixing time for each solution.

2. Create a discontinuous gradient by first placing 3 mL of the 5% iodixanol solution to the bottom of the centrifuge tube with a long blunt end needle. Subsequently, underlay 3 mL of the 10% iodixanol, followed by 3 mL of the 20% iodixanol (*see* **Note 9**).

3. Place 3 mL of the 40% iodixanol solution containing nanoparticles from Subheading 3.2, **step 6** at the bottom of the discontinuous gradient.

4. After balancing the tubes within 0.1 g of each other, centrifuge in an SW 40 Ti rotor at $100,000 \times g$ for 18 h in Optima XPN 90 ultracentrifuge.

5. After centrifugation, gently collect 12 individual 1 mL fractions from the top of the tubes.

3.4 Fraction Density Determination (See Note 10)

1. Add 100 μL of the 5%, 10%, and 20% iodixanol standards along with each of the fractions into 100 μL of water in a 96-well plate. Subject the samples to thorough mixing by pipetting up and down three times. Perform each measurement in triplicate.

2. Measure the absorbance of the individual solutions in each well using a plate reader containing a 340 nm filter.

Table 1
Iodixanol gradient solutions for exosome isolation

Iodixanol solutions, w/v (%)	50% Iodixanol, w/v (mL)	Homogenization buffer (mL)	Total (mL)	Density (g/mL)
5	2	18	20	1.054
10	4	16	20	1.079
20	8	12	20	1.127

3. Create a standard curve by plotting the densities of the 5%, 10%, and 20% iodixanol solutions (Table 1) against the mean absorbance.

4. Use the mean absorbance of each fraction to calculate the density of each fraction from the standard curve.

3.5 Protein Quantification by Qubit Protein Assay

1. Label three tubes for the standards and one tube for each fraction.

2. Prepare Qubit Working Solution by diluting the Qubit Protein Reagent 1:200 in Qubit Protein Buffer.

3. Add 190 μL Qubit working solution and 10 μL standards or samples into the corresponding assay tube.

4. Vortex standards and samples for 2–3 s and incubate at room temperature for 15 min.

5. Select Protein Assay on the Qubit 3.0 Fluorometer to calibrate with standards and read the samples.

3.6 Protein Characterization by SDS-PAGE and Immunoblotting

1. Mix 90 μL of each fraction with 10 μL of 10× RIPA buffer, PMSF, and Laemmli buffer. Boil the mixed samples at 95 °C for 5 min.

2. Prepare 10% polyacrylamide gels containing SDS as a denaturant.

3. Load the gels with a molecular-weight marker spanning 10 kDa to 250 kDa along with the denatured samples and resolve the proteins by electrophoresis.

4. Visualization of resolved proteins in the PAGE is achieved by incubating the gel with Coomassie stain for 2 h.

5. Subsequently, the gels are destained in 5% methanol and 7.5% glacial acetic acid solution and images are captured using an ImageQuant LAS 4000.

6. For western blot detection, transfer proteins resolved in the PAGE onto nitrocellulose membranes using a standard western blot transfer protocol.

7. Block the unbound sites within the membrane with 5% non-fat milk for 1 h at room temperature.

8. Immunostain proteins with anti-TSG101 antibody (1:200) and anti-Alix antibody (1:1000) diluted in 5% non-fat milk and agitate membranes overnight at 4 °C.

9. Wash membranes for 5 min four times at room temperature with 1× PBST.

10. Incubate membranes with IRDye 680RD Goat anti-Mouse IgG (1:15,000) and IRDye 800CW Goat anti-Rabbit IgG (1:15,000) in 5% non-fat milk for 1 h at room temperature. Protect membranes from light starting at this step.

11. Wash membranes for 5 min four times at room temperature with 1× PBST in the dark. Rinse membranes twice with D-PBS.

12. Scan membranes with Odyssey Infrared Imaging System at 700 and 800 nm.

13. Determine the presence of exosome markers in the iodixanol gradient fractions.

3.7 Exosome Characterization by Flow Cytometry

1. Incubate 10 µg purified exosomes with 10 µL latex beads for 15 min at room temperature in a 1.5-mL Eppendorf tube with continuous rotation.

2. Add 1 mL D-PBS and incubate 4 °C overnight with continuous rotation.

3. Add 110 µL of 1 M glycine (i.e., 100 mM final), mix gently, and incubate at room temperature for 30 min.

4. Pellet the beads at 5000×*g* for 3 min at room temperature, remove the supernatant and discard.

5. Resuspend the pellet in 1 mL D-PBS/0.5% BSA, and re-pellet the beads at 4000 rpm for 3 min, remove the supernatant and discard.

6. Resuspend beads in 0.5 mL D-PBS /0.5% BSA.

7. Incubate 10 µL coated beads with 10 µL anti-exosomal protein antibody diluted in D-PBS/0.5% BSA 30 min at 4 °C.

8. Wash twice with 1 mL D-PBS/0.5% BSA.

9. Add 200 µL of D-PBS/0.5% BSA and analyze the beads by flow cytometry.

3.8 Exosome Enumeration by Nanoparticle Tracking Analysis

1. Identify the optimal region in LM14 Nanosight for video capture; flush the chamber with 2 mL pure water (*see* **Note 11**).

2. Dilute the exosome samples with pure water to create 1 mL of solution at an optimal concentration (*see* **Note 12**).

3. Aspirate the exosome sample into a 1 mL syringe and infuse 0.5 mL into the sample chamber, taking care to ensure that no air bubbles are introduced to the system.

4. Fine tune to refocus the particles and set the infusion rate at 40.

5. Set appropriate camera level and screen gain, record three videos, 1 min each.

6. Set appropriate detection level and analyze the captured video files.

3.9 Exosomal RNA Extraction

1. Add 400 µL exosome sample in 2 mL tubes.

2. Add 400 µL pre-warmed 2× Denaturing Solution. Immediately mix thoroughly.

3. Add 800 µL of the bottom phase of Acid-Phenol:Chloroform.

4. Vortex for 30–60 s to mix.

5. Centrifuge for 5 min at 14,000 × g at room temperature to separate the mixture into aqueous and organic phases.

6. Carefully remove the aqueous (upper) phase without disturbing the lower phase or the interphase, and transfer it to a fresh tube.

7. Add 1.25 volumes of 100% ethanol to the aqueous phase and mix thoroughly.

8. For each sample, place a filter cartridge into one of the collection tubes.

9. Pipet the lysate/ethanol mixture onto the filter cartridge. Apply a maximum of 700 μL to a filter cartridge at a time.

10. Centrifuge at 10,000 × g for ~30 s.

11. Discard the flow-through, and repeat until all of the lysate/ethanol mixture is through the filter. Save the collection tube for the washing steps.

12. Apply 700 μL miRNA Wash Solution 1 to the Filter Cartridge and centrifuge at 10,000 × g for ~15 s, discard the flow-through from the collection tube, and replace the filter cartridge into the same collection tube.

13. Apply 500 μL Wash Solution 2/3 and draw it through the Filter Cartridge as in the previous step.

14. Repeat with a second 500 μL of Wash Solution 2/3.

15. After discarding the flow-through from the last wash, replace the filter cartridge in the same collection tube and spin the assembly for 1 min at to remove residual fluid from the filter.

16. Transfer the filter cartridge into a fresh collection tube. Apply 50 μL of preheated (95 °C) nuclease-free water to the center of the filter, and close the cap. Centrifuge for ~30 s to recover the RNA.

17. Collect the eluate and store it at −80 °C.

3.10 Exosomal Total RNA Characterization

1. Using an Agilent 2100 Bioanalyzer system, prepare a Gel-Dye mix by mixing 1 μL RNA dye concentrate with 65 μL filtered gel, vortex solution well, and spin the tube at 13,000 × g for 10 min at room temperature.

2. Load 9 μL Gel-Dye mix to appropriate well and prime the RNA Pico chip.

3. Load 9 μL Gel-Dye mix and the RNA conditioning solution to appropriate well.

4. Pipet 5 μL of RNA marker in the well for ladder and all 11 sample wells.

5. Pipet 1 μL of the heat denatured ladder into the ladder well.

6. Pipet 1 μL of sample in each of the 11 sample wells.

7. Vortex for 1 min at 2400 rpm in the IKA station.

8. Run the chip in the Agilent 2100 Bioanalyzer within 5 min.

3.11 Exosomal Small RNA Characterization

1. Prepare the Gel-Dye mixture by combining the RNA dye concentrate with filtered gel, vortex the solution well, and spin the tube at $13,000 \times g$ for 10 min at room temperature.

2. Load 9 µL Gel-Dye mix to appropriate well and prime the small RNA chip.

3. Load 9 µL Gel-Dye mix and the RNA conditioning solution to appropriate wells.

4. Pipet 5 µL of RNA marker in the well for ladder and all 11 sample wells.

5. Pipet 1 µL of the heat denatured ladder into the ladder well.

6. Pipet 1 µL of sample in each of the 11 sample wells.

7. Vortex for 1 min at 2400 rpm in the IKA station.

8. Run the chip in the Agilent 2100 Bioanalyzer within 5 min.

4 Notes

1. Standard Fetal Bovine Serum (FBS) contains very high levels of bovine extracellular vesicles and lipoproteins which will complicate downstream analyses if not thoroughly removed prior to use for cell culture. It is therefore important to eliminate these native nanoparticles by an overnight centrifugation at $100,000 \times g$.

2. The use of Iodixanol offers several advantages over sucrose. First, solutions of iodixanol display lower viscosity than sucrose solutions, making it easier to handle. Second, iodixanol is thought to be metabolically inert and nontoxic to cells, allowing subsequent functional assays to be performed without the need for its removal which can, however, be achieved through dialysis. Lastly, Iodixanol solutions also display lower osmolality than sucrose solutions at similar density and can be made iso-osmotic at high densities, allowing exosomes to be purified under iso-osmotic conditions and thus better preserve their integrity and functionality.

3. It is recommended to prepare a 50% iodixanol stock solution, which makes it easier than 60% iodixanol to create 5%, 10%, and 20% iodixanol solutions. To prepare a 50% iodixanol stock, mix 5 volumes of OptiPrep with 1 volume of 1.5 M sucrose, 6 mM EDTA, 60 mM Tris–HCl, pH 7.4. On standing, iodixanol tends to settle; always shake the bottle of OptiPrep to obtain a homogeneous solution before use.

4. Swinging-bucket rotors are advantageous over fixed-angle rotors for gradient work since the gradient always maintains

the same orientation with the axis of the tube and the longer path length permits better separation of exosomes.

5. Cells, cellular debris, and other large microparticles are first removed from the conditioned medium by differential centrifugation and filtration. Omission of these clarification steps may lead to a loss of exosomes due to their entrapment into aggregates that rapidly form and sediment as large particles at high centrifugal force.

6. The yields of exosomes vary considerably depending on cell type and culture condition. A larger volume of conditioned media may be required for some downstream experiments, such as western blot protein detection and RNA sequencing. Ultrafiltration devices, e.g., Amicon Ultra-15 centrifugal filters, can be used for concentrating exosomes from conditioned media before ultracentrifugation.

7. Iodixanol solutions tend to adhere to the walls of a pipette, making it difficult to accurately transfer with pipetting. The use of syringes is therefore recommended for accurate dispensing. It is best to take up more of iodixanol medium than is required as it is more accurate to empty the syringe to a graduation mark than to empty it completely.

8. At a given centrifugal g-force, the time required for complete sedimentation of vesicles largely depends on the path length of the rotor. As swinging-bucket rotors have a greater path length than fixed-angle rotors, the run time for swinging-bucket rotors will be longer for efficient sedimentation.

9. A convenient way to create discontinuous gradients is by underlaying successively denser solutions beneath lighter ones. A syringe fitted with a metal filling cannula is an ideal tool for this procedure. Add 10% or 20% solutions very slowly to avoid mixing with 5% or 10% solutions, respectively. It is also important to avoid air bubble formation during dispensing, as it will disturb the lower density layers.

10. Density analysis can be simply performed by measuring the absorbance at 340 nm on gradient fractions using multi-well plate readers. However, because there is a linear relationship between refractive index and density, the solutions density can also be determined by measuring the refractive index of the gradient fraction if a wide-range Refractometer is available.

11. Nanoparticles are present in many commercially available buffers. It is important to test if the buffer is free of particles prior to its use.

12. Accurate quantification of exosomes and other nanoparticles using NTA works best when sample concentrations are between 10^8 and 10^9 particles per mL of solution. An optimum dilution would present around 100 particles in the field of view when inserted into the sample chamber and visualized.

Acknowledgments

This work was supported by grants from the American Heart Association (16GRNT27640007), National Institutes of Health; (5U19CA179512) Extracellular RNA Communication Consortium Common Fund, and HL133575 to (R.L.R.) which was administered by the Northern California Institute for Research and Education. The work was performed at the Veterans Affairs Medical Center, San Francisco, CA.

References

1. Colombo M, Raposo G, Thery C (2014) Biogenesis, secretion, and intercellular interactions of exosomes and other extracellular vesicles. Annu Rev Cell Dev Biol 30:255–289

2. Valadi H, Ekstrom K, Bossios A, Sjostrand M, Lee JJ, Lotvall JO (2007) Exosome-mediated transfer of mRNAs and microRNAs is a novel mechanism of genetic exchange between cells. Nat Cell Biol 9:654–659

3. Yanez-Mo M, Siljander PR, Andreu Z, Zavec AB, Borras FE, Buzas EI, Buzas K, Casal E, Cappello F, Carvalho J et al (2015) Biological properties of extracellular vesicles and their physiological functions. J Extracell Vesicles 4:27066

4. Gyorgy B, Hung ME, Breakefield XO, Leonard JN (2015) Therapeutic applications of extracellular vesicles: clinical promise and open questions. Annu Rev Pharmacol Toxicol 55:439–464

5. Kourembanas S (2015) Exosomes: vehicles of intercellular signaling, biomarkers, and vectors of cell therapy. Annu Rev Physiol 77:13–27

6. Johnstone RM, Adam M, Hammond JR, Orr L, Turbide C (1987) Vesicle formation during reticulocyte maturation. Association of plasma membrane activities with released vesicles (exosomes). J Biol Chem 262:9412–9420

7. Thery C, Amigorena S, Raposo G, Clayton A (2006) Isolation and characterization of exosomes from cell culture supernatants and biological fluids. Curr Protoc Cell Biol. Chapter 3:Unit 3.22

8. Linares R, Tan S, Gounou C, Arraud N, Brisson AR (2015) High-speed centrifugation induces aggregation of extracellular vesicles. J Extracell Vesicles 4:29509

9. Momen-Heravi F, Balaj L, Alian S, Mantel PY, Halleck AE, Trachtenberg AJ, Soria CE, Oquin S, Bonebreak CM, Saracoglu E et al (2013) Current methods for the isolation of extracellular vesicles. Biol Chem 394:1253–1262

10. Nordin JZ, Lee Y, Vader P, Mager I, Johansson HJ, Heusermann W, Wiklander OP, Hallbrink M, Seow Y, Bultema JJ et al (2015) Ultrafiltration with size-exclusion liquid chromatography for high yield isolation of extracellular vesicles preserving intact biophysical and functional properties. Nanomedicine 11:879–883

11. Abramowicz A, Widlak P, Pietrowska M (2016) Proteomic analysis of exosomal cargo: the challenge of high purity vesicle isolation. Mol Biosyst 12:1407–1419

12. Van Deun J, Mestdagh P, Agostinis P, Akay O, Anand S, Anckaert J, Martinez ZA, Baetens T, Beghein E, Bertier L et al (2017) EV-TRACK: transparent reporting and centralizing knowledge in extracellular vesicle research. Nat Methods 14:228–232

13. Elmowalid GA, Qiao M, Jeong SH, Borg BB, Baumert TF, Sapp RK, Hu Z, Murthy K, Liang TJ (2007) Immunization with hepatitis C virus-like particles results in control of hepatitis C virus infection in chimpanzees. Proc Natl Acad Sci U S A 104:8427–8432

14. Greening DW, Xu R, Ji H, Tauro BJ, Simpson RJ (2015) A protocol for exosome isolation and characterization: evaluation of ultracentrifugation, density-gradient separation, and immunoaffinity capture methods. Methods Mol Biol 1295:179–209

15. Lamparski HG, Metha-Damani A, Yao JY, Patel S, Hsu DH, Ruegg C, Le Pecq JB (2002) Production and characterization of clinical grade exosomes derived from dendritic cells. J Immunol Methods 270:211–226

16. Lobb RJ, Becker M, Wen SW, Wong CS, Wiegmans AP, Leimgruber A, Moller A (2015) Optimized exosome isolation protocol for cell culture supernatant and human plasma. J Extracell Vesicles 4:27031

Chapter 8

Magnetic Particle-Based Immunoprecipitation of Nanoscale Extracellular Vesicles from Biofluids

Pete Heinzelman

Abstract

Analysis of nanoscale extracellular vesicles (nsEVs) present in blood, cell culture media, and other biofluids has shown tremendous promise in enabling the development of noninvasive blood-based clinical diagnostic tests, predicting and monitoring the efficacy of treatment programs, and providing molecular level insights into pathology that can enlighten new drug targets in the contexts of health conditions such as cancer and Alzheimer's Disease (AD). In this chapter, we present methods for using magnetic particle-based immunoprecipitation to enrich highly purified populations of nsEVs directly from plasma, serum, and other biofluids. These methods enable downstream analysis of nsEV protein and nucleic acid constituents in the contexts of both global omics profiling and quantification of individual protein or nucleic acid species of interest. Additionally, these methods allow the researcher to either enrich total nsEV populations or enrich nsEVs derived from a particular tissue type from the overall nsEV population. The methods described here are compatible with parallel processing of dozens of biofluid samples and can be valuable tools for enabling nsEV analyses that have high translational relevance in the development of both novel therapeutics and noninvasive diagnostic assays.

Key words Proteomics, Extracellular vesicle, Exosome, Ultracentrifugation, Diagnostics, Liquid biopsy, Immunoprecipitation, Transcriptomics, Next-generation sequencing

1 Introduction

Nanoscale extracellular vesicles (nsEVs), which we define as spherical particles with submicron diameters that either bud off from cell plasma membranes (ectosomes) or are secreted by cells after formation within cytoplasmic multivesicular bodies (exosomes), can inform molecular level changes associated with disease onset and progression via two mechanisms [1]. First, given that nsEVs carry signaling molecules, in particular proteins and nucleic acids that transmit information from one cell to another, differences in nsEV composition across normal and diseased subjects can reflect changes in intercellular communication that either contribute to or are the result of disease pathology. Second, as the contents of nsEVs mirror the content of the cells from which they originate,

Tushar Patel (ed.), *Extracellular RNA: Methods and Protocols*, Methods in Molecular Biology, vol. 1740,
https://doi.org/10.1007/978-1-4939-7652-2_8, © Springer Science+Business Media, LLC 2018

disease-associated differences in nsEV composition relative to normal nsEVs can be indicators of protein or nucleic acid abundance changes that either promote or are by-products of the disease state.

Obtaining tissue samples for clinical diagnostic tests often requires invasive biopsy procedures and is especially problematic in seeking to diagnose diseases of the central nervous system (CNS) due to the risks and high cost associated with craniotomy. In contrast, adequate numbers of nsEVs for diagnostic tests can be isolated from microliter volumes of blood obtained during a routine draw that is readily performed during a doctor's office visit. This ease of isolation has motivated the development of blood-borne nsEV-based assays for diagnosing several types of cancer [2, 3] and also CNS disorders including Alzheimer's Disease (AD) [4–7] and Parkinson's Disease (PD) [8]. The observation that changes in the abundances of blood-borne nsEV biomarker proteins can accurately predict the onset of AD up to 10 years prior to clinical manifestation of symptoms is a particularly impressive result in this still burgeoning research area [4].

In addition to the still largely unrealized potential of blood-borne nsEv analysis in facilitating the development of noninvasive clinical diagnostic assays, characterization of nsEVs isolated from both corporeal biofluids, such as blood and saliva, and in vitro disease tissue culture model culture media supernatant offers an exciting opportunity to enlighten changes in cellular signaling mechanisms and biochemistry that underlie disease onset and progression. This knowledge can find great translational relevance in both leading to the identification of new drug targets and the development of new treatment paradigms that are based on existing drugs and/or new therapeutic molecules.

Many of the methods used, such as ultracentrifugation (UC) and chemical precipitation (CP), for enriching nsEVs for proteomic analysis [9], next-generation nucleic acid sequencing (NGS) [10], or quantification of individual nsEV protein [4] or nucleic acid species [11] isolate not only nsEVs but also high levels of contaminants including albumin, IgGs, lipoprotein complexes, and debris originating from dead cells [12–14]. The presence of these contaminants, which tend to be more abundant in preparations of nsEVs enriched from corporeal biofluids than in preparations enriched from cell culture media, can present challenges to accurately quantifying nsEV constituents in the contexts of all of the nsEV molecular constituent characterization procedures noted above.

The appearance of high intensity background signals, caused by contaminants in nsEV preparations, during mass spectrometric profiling of nsEv proteomes can both impede reliable quantification of differences in nsEV protein abundances across nsEV samples obtained from different biofluid specimens, e.g., pools of plasma from respective diseased and normal patient groups, and preclude the detection of low abundance nsEV proteome constituents [15].

Contaminants in nsEV preparations can also reduce the fidelity of assays, e.g., enzyme-linked immunosorbent assay (ELISA) or bead-based immunofluorescence assays, used to measure abundances of individual or selected small groups of nsEV protein constituents. The observation that levels of cytokines in adipose stem cell culture media nsEV preparations, as measured by a multiplex bead-based Luminex assay [16], were up to 100-fold greater for PBS washed nsEV preparations isolated via UC than for unwashed nsEV preparations enriched using UC is a compelling example of how contaminants can skew nsEV protein constituent quantification datasets.

In addition to compromising the quality of data obtained in both proteomic profiling studies and individual nsEV protein constituent measurement assays contaminants in nsEV preparations may preclude accurate identification and/or quantification of nsEV nucleic acid molecules. Lipoprotein complexes, which are abundant in plasma and are often co-enriched with nsEVs during nsEV isolation, are known to carry microRNAs (miRNAs) that can preclude both accurate quantification of individual nsEV miRNAs using qRT-PCR and reliable characterization of nsEV miRNA transcriptomes via NGS [10]. Furthermore, the presence of cell-free DNA, which may be present at relatively high concentrations in biofluids that are in contact with or contain abnormally large numbers of apoptotic or necrotic cells [17] and like lipoprotein complexes has been observed to co-enrich with nsEVs [10], in nsEV preparations can preclude the use of spectrophotometric or fluorescent dye-based assays to determine the total RNA content of nsEV preparations [10] and thus make it challenging to accurately compare abundances of individual nsEV ribonucleic acids in nsEV preparations derived from different biofluid specimens.

The challenge of preventing nsEV preparation contaminants from compromising the quality of nsEV characterization data can be addressed by using magnetic particle-based immunoprecipitation (IP) to isolate nsEVs from biofluid specimens. Such IP procedures, which employ antibody (Ab)-coupled magnetic particles, e.g., Dynabeads (ThermoFisher Scientific), that bind to generic nsEV surface marker proteins such as the tetraspanin proteins CD9, CD63, and CD81 or tissue-specific nsEV surface marker proteins such as CD56 or CD171 for neurons [4], yield nsEV preparations with markedly higher purity than those obtained by using CP or UC procedures. These IP protocols are compatible with parallel processing of multiple biofluid specimens and require only minimal processing, i.e., simple centrifugation and syringe filtration, of biofluid specimens prior to nsEV precipitation (Fig. 1).

The multivalent nature of the Dynabeads-nsEV binding interaction gives rise to an avidity effect [18] that allows one to carry out high stringency, i.e., aqueous buffer with a pH below 3, washes without causing excessive dissociation of nsEVs from the Ab-coupled Dynabeads. These high stringency washes, which

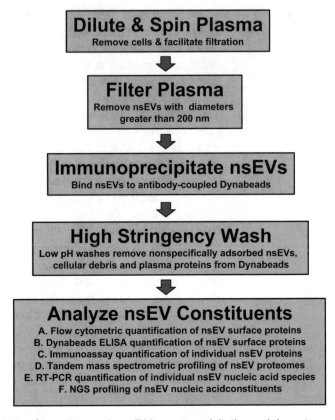

Fig. 1 Block flow diagram for nsEV immunoprecipitation and downstream characterization of nsEV protein and nucleic acid constituents

remove nonspecifically bound entities, i.e., the contaminants enumerated above, are key in enabling the enrichment of high purity cell culture media, plasma, or serum nsEV populations. Although we are not aware of cases in which such high stringency washes have been used in the context of IP of nsEVs from homogenized solid tissue samples [19], it is probable that these stringent low pH wash conditions would enable nsEVs residing within homogenized tissue specimens to be enriched to high purity.

In addition to detailing the Dynabeads-based methods for IP of high purity nsEV populations from biofluids that have been alluded to above this chapter presents methods for using both flow cytometry and colorimetric ELISA to quantify levels of proteins presented on the surfaces of Dynabeads-bound nsEVs [20]. This chapter also offers guidance in terms of utilizing nsEV IP as a lead-in to subsequent shotgun tandem mass spectrometric profiling of nsEV proteomes [21], measurement of individual nsEV protein constituent levels using ELISAs or fluorescent immunoassays, quantification of nsEV nucleic acid constituents using qRT-PCR, and omics level nsEV nucleic acid analysis via NGS. Taken together, the methods and guidance presented in this chapter comprise a body of information that can markedly enhance the fidelity with which researchers can identify and quantify nsEV protein and nucleic acid constituents. This enhancement can play an important role in enabling those working in this still relatively nascent research field to maximally realize the exciting potential to leverage nsEV analysis in developing both novel therapeutics and noninvasive diagnostic assays that can improve patient outcomes and enlighten preventative strategies across a wide range of health conditions.

2   Materials

2.1   Clearance of Plasma for Immunoprecipitation

1. Water bath.
2. Benchtop vortexer.
3. Refrigerated microcentrifuge.
4. Low binding 1.5 mL microfuge tubes. Appropriate low binding tubes are available from a number of suppliers, such as ThermoFisher Scientific (Grand Island, NY) and Eppendorf (Hauppauge, NY), and should be used throughout the methods described in this chapter to prevent nsEVs, Dynabeads, and proteins and/or nucleic acids in nsEV extracts from becoming nonspecifically adsorbed on plasticware surfaces.
5. Filtered (0.2 μm) phosphate buffered saline (PBS), pH 7.4.
6. AcroVac PES membrane (0.2 μm pore size) filter units (Pall Life Sciences, Port Washington, NY).
7. Disposable Luer-lok plastic syringes.
8. Supor membrane (0.2 μm pore size) PES syringe filters (Pall Life Sciences).
9. Halt protease/phosphatase inhibitor cocktail (ThermoFisher Scientific).

2.2   nsEV Immunoprecipitation from Plasma

1. DynaMag-2 (ThermoFisher Scientific, Grand Island, NY).
2. Benchtop minifuge.
3. Hula mixer (ThermoFisher Scientific).
4. Benchtop vortexer.
5. Dynabeads CD63 Exosome Isolation/Detection Reagent, CD9 Exosome Isolation Reagent or CD81 Exosome Isolation Reagent, or Dynabeads Antibody Coupling Kit; this kit contains Dynabeads M-270 Epoxy (ThermoFisher Scientific).
6. Abs for coupling to Dynabeads Epoxy as appropriate.
7. Molecular biology grade bovine serum albumin (BSA), ≥98% pure.
8. Low pH IgG elution buffer (ThermoFisher Scientific).

9. PBS containing 0.1% (w/v) BSA [PBSA]: Dissolve 1 g of BSA in 1 L of PBS and vacuum filter through 0.2 μm PES membrane filter unit (Subheading 2.1, **item 6** above).

10. PBS containing 1% (w/v) BSA [PBSW]: Dissolve 10 g of BSA in 1 L of PBS and vacuum filter through 0.2 μm PES membrane filter unit.

11. 25 mM phosphate-citrate buffer, pH 5.0: Add 2.35 g citric acid and 4.6 g $Na_2HPO_4 \cdot 2H_2O$ (Dibasic Sodium Phosphate Dihydrate) to 1 L of deionized water, adjust pH to 5.0, and vacuum filter through 0.2 μM PES membrane.

12. Molecular biology grade Tween-20.

2.3 Flow Cytometric Quantification of Surface Proteins Presented by Magnetic Particle-Bound nsEVs

1. Flow cytometer featuring appropriate laser and detection filters for phycoerythrin (PE) excitation and PE fluorescence measurement.

2. Benchtop vortex mixer.

3. Biotinylated, PE-conjugated, or unconjugated Abs-binding nsEV surface protein(s) of interest.

4. Isotype-matched negative control Abs.

5. EZ-Link Sulfo-NHS-LC-Biotin for Ab biotinylation as appropriate (ThermoFisher Scientific).

6. PE-conjugated streptavidin: Dissolve lyophilized protein powder (Jackson ImmunoResearch, West Grove, PA) at 1 mg/mL in sterile H_2O and store in aliquots at −20 °C for use as secondary label in conjunction with biotinylated anti-nsEV surface protein Abs.

7. Appropriate plastic tubes for loading cytometry samples onto flow cytometer used for analysis.

8. PBSA.

9. PBSW.

10. PBS containing 2.5% (w/v) BSA [PBSL]: Dissolve 25 g of BSA in 1 L of PBS and vacuum filter through 0.2 μm PES membrane filter unit.

2.4 Magnetic Particle ELISA Colorimetric Quantification of Surface Proteins Presented by Magnetic Particle-Bound nsEVs

1. 96-Well platereader capable of measuring absorbance at 450 nm.

2. Benchtop vortex mixer.

3. Biotinylated or unconjugated Abs-binding nsEV surface protein(s) of interest.

4. Isotype-matched negative control Abs.

5. EZ-Link Sulfo-NHS-LC-Biotin for Ab biotinylation as appropriate (ThermoFisher Scientific).

6. Horseradish peroxidase (HRP)-conjugated streptavidin: Dissolve lyophilized protein powder (Jackson ImmunoResearch) at 1 mg/mL in sterile H_2O and store in aliquots at -20 °C for use as secondary label in conjunction with biotinylated anti-nsEV surface protein Abs.

7. 96-well transparent flat bottom microplates.

8. PBSA.

9. PBSW.

10. PBSL.

11. 2 N Sulfuric acid.

12. One-Step UltraTMB (3,3′,5,5′-Tetramethylbenzidine) ELISA substrate (ThermoFisher Scientific).

2.5 Quantification of Magnetic Particle-Immunoprecipitated nsEV Protein Constituents

1. Materials for nsEV protein constituent shogun proteomic profiling are described at length elsewhere [21].

2. For quantification of individual or small sets of nsEV protein constituents required apparatuses, reagents and/or kits are determined by the researcher based on the protein quantification methods being employed.

2.6 Quantification of Magnetic Particle-Immunoprecipitated nsEV Nucleic Acid Constituents

1. Qiagen MicroRNA Easy kit (Qiagen, Orange, CA).

2. RiboGreen RNA assay kit (ThermoFisher Scientific).

3. Nucleic acid amplification and analysis apparatuses, qRT-PCR reagents, and amplification reaction primers or RNA library construction kits based on nsEV nucleic acid characterizations to be performed by the researcher.

3 Methods

The procedures for obtaining highly purified nsEVs from serum, plasma, cell culture media supernatant, or other biofluids require two partial days of labor. Preparation of biofluid samples for IP on day 1 requires approximately 2 h. After overnight incubation of Ab-coupled Dynabeads with biofluid specimens, approximately 1 h of processing is required to obtain highly purified nsEVs; these nsEVs are tightly bound to Dynabeads via multivalent interactions with anti-nsEV surface marker Abs that have been covalently coupled to Dynabeads surfaces either by the manufacturer, e.g., Dynabeads CD81 Exosome Isolation Reagent, or the researcher, i.e., manual coupling of Ab of interest to Dynabeads M-270 Epoxy. Both flow cytometric [20] and ELISA assays can be used to quantify relative abundances of nsEV surface proteins presented by the nsEVs that are bound by the Dynabeads-coupled anti-nsEV surface marker protein Abs. Alternatively, one can employ nsEV lysis methods, such as exposure to detergents [4–8, 21], to enable subsequent extraction and isolation of nsEV protein and/or nucleic acid constituents for subsequent downstream omics profiling and/or quantification of individual nsEV biomolecular constituents using approaches such as high sensitivity fluorescent immunoassays [8, 22] or qRT-PCR [23].

As the author has more extensive experience isolating nsEVs from plasma and serum than from other biofluids this chapter describes methods for isolation and downstream analysis of nsEVs present within these blood-derived biofluids. Regardless of this chapter's focus on plasma and serum specimens minor adaptations to the methods presented have enabled isolation of nsEVs from saliva, cerebrospinal fluid, and cell culture media supernatant.

Adjustment of biofluid specimen dilution factors prior to IP to account for differences in biofluid viscosity [24] and increasing the specimen volume:Dynabeads ratio to account for the low per unit volume nsEV concentrations of some biofluids, such as cerebrospinal fluid [25], relative to blood-derived biofluids are the modifications that have most frequently been made in applying the methods of this chapter to isolation of nsEVs from biofluids other than plasma and serum. Combining the procedures detailed below with an awareness of the potential need for such adjustments positions, the researcher to enrich highly purified populations of nsEVs from essentially any biofluid of interest and achieve high fidelity identification and quantification of nsEV protein and/or nucleic acid constituents.

3.1 Clearance of Plasma or Serum for Immunoprecipitation

1. This protocol is compatible with either fresh or freeze-thawed plasma or serum. We recommend using plasma or serum samples that have been prepared using EDTA as coagulant and that have not been put through more than one freeze-thaw cycle.

2. For frozen samples, thaw in a 37 °C water bath until the last crystals of ice in the tubes have just disappeared. After thawing is complete, mix the samples by gently vortexing for 10 s. All handling steps from this point forward should be carried out on ice or in a refrigerated centrifuge.

3. Dilute plasma 1:1.5 with PBS, i.e., add 500 μL of PBS to 1 mL of plasma and mix by gently vortexing as above. Pending the volume of each plasma sample aliquot into 1.5 mL low bind microcentrifuge tubes on ice and spin at 4 °C for 20 min at 13,000 rcf.

4. Depending on the volume of each plasma sample, prewet either a 13 mm diameter 0.2 μm PES syringe filter (used for sample volumes of 1 mL or less) or a 25 mm diameter PES syringe filter by passing 2 mL of PBS through the filter. We recommend using 3 mL disposable plastic syringes for 13 mm

diameter filters and 10 mL disposable plastic syringes for 25 mm diameter filters. A separate filter and syringe should be used for each sample being filtered.

5. After the above centrifugation step, there will be a pellet at the bottom of the tube and most probably also a layer of solid material floating on top of the liquid. Remove the supernatant from the tubes while taking care to minimize the amount of solid floating material that is drawn up with the liquid. Add Halt protease/phosphatase inhibitor cocktail to the supernatant at a 1:50 volumetric dilution ratio; this is twice the manufacturer's recommended concentration. Carefully pass the plasma specimens through the prewetted syringe filters while taking care to minimize sample foaming.

6. Filtered samples can be stored on ice until Dynabeads have been prepared for the IP procedure.

3.2 Preparing Magnetic Particles for nsEV Immunoprecipitation from Plasma

1. Although the IP method detailed in this chapter (Fig. 1) is likely to be compatible with other magnetic particles, the procedures described have been optimized for Dynabeads Exosome Isolation magnetic particle products for cases in which one wishes to immunoprecipitate total nsEV populations. For isolation of nsEVs presenting a tissue-type marker, such as CD56 or CD171 for neuronal nsEVs, the IP procedure has been optimized for Dynabeads M-270 Epoxy covalently coupled (*see* **Note 1**) with the anti-tissue type marker mAb of interest using the protocol described below. The researcher may also prepare Dynabeads Epoxy coupled with Abs that bind generic nsEV surface protein markers, such as CD63 and CD81, as an alternative to using the pre-coupled Dynabeads Exosome Isolation products enumerated in Subheading 2.2, **item 2** above.

2. Abs have generally been coupled to Dynabeads M-270 Epoxy in 5 mg batches per a slightly modified version of the manufacturer's protocol. With respect to this modification, the manufacturer's recommended washing steps are preceded by a 10-min incubation, with tumbling on a lab mixer, of Dynabeads in low pH (pH less than 3) buffer such as glycine-HCl or IgG elution buffer (*see* **Note 2**).

3. For each mL of diluted plasma IP should be carried out with 200 μL of Dynabeads CD63 Exosome Isolation/Detection Reagent (~10^7 particles/mL as packaged), 20 μL CD9 Exosome Isolation Reagent (~10^8 particles/mL as packaged), 20 μL CD81 Exosome Isolation Reagent (~10^8 particles/mL as packaged), or 5 μL of Ab-coupled Dynabeads M-270 Epoxy (resuspended at ~6.7×10^8 particles/mL, *see* **Notes 3** and **4**). Block Dynabeads by adding to 750 μL of ice cold PBSA in a microcentrifuge tube and allowing to gently rotate on an

appropriate tube mixer, such as a Hula Mixer, at 4 °C for 1 h. Adjust mixer settings so that buffer foaming does not occur; foaming may occur if head-over-head tube mixing is employed.

4. Apply a magnet, such as the DynaMag2, to draw the Dynabeads to the side of the tube and remove the PBSA with a pipette.

5. Pending sample volumes add up to 1.2 mL of diluted, filtered plasma directly to the blocked Dynabeads and mix by gently vortexing.

6. Incubate Dynabeads with plasma overnight (16–24 h) on a tube mixer at 4 °C (*see* **Note 5**).

7. Remove microfuge tubes from the lab rotator and spin in a benchtop minifuge for 10 s. Apply magnet to draw the Dynabeads to the side of the tube. Slowly withdraw the nsEV-depleted plasma without drawing any Dynabeads into the pipette with the plasma. It is important to remove all of the plasma from the microcentrifuge tube. The Dynabeads will form a vertical streak along the side of the tube.

8. Immunoprecipitation is followed by four washes: 1 min without tube rotation in PBSA, 10 min with rotation on a lab mixer in the low pH buffer noted above (*see* **Note 6**), a repeat of this low pH wash step, and a final 1-min wash in PBSA. Between each wash step magnetic microspheres are drawn to the side of the 1.5 mL microcentrifuge tubes in which all incubations are carried out using a DynaMag and the wash supernatant is removed by pipetting. Five-hundred microliters of wash buffer are used for each wash step.

9. After completing the final wash step, IPed nsEV protein and/ or nucleic acid constituents can be analyzed using the methods described in Subheadings 3.3–3.6 (*see* **Notes 7** and **8**) or via other procedures that the reader may wish to employ based on their experience and nsEV constituent characterization needs.

3.3 Flow Cytometric Quantification of Surface Proteins Presented by Magnetic Particle-Bound nsEVs

1. Abs binding to epitopes presented by proteins, such as tetraspanins or tissue-type marker proteins CD56 and CD171, on nsEV membrane exteriors can be used to quantify nsEV surface proteins using either flow cytometry or a magnetic particle ELISA assay that is described below in Subheading 3.4. In both cases, nsEV surface protein detection Abs are incubated with Dynabeads-nsEV complexes (Fig. 2) following nsEV IP and washing of Dynabeads as discussed in Subheading 3.2. Flow cytometric detection may be carried out using either biotinylated anti-nsEV surface protein Abs as primary labeling agents followed by secondary labeling with fluorescent streptavidin or fluorescently conjugated anti-nsEV surface protein Abs (*see* **Note 9**).

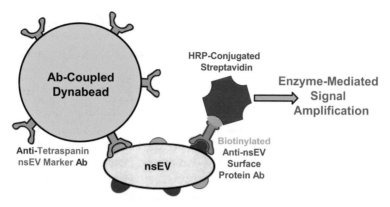

Fig. 2 Dynabeads-nsEV IP and flow cytometric nsEV surface protein quantification schematic. The researcher is free to couple any Ab of interest (figure depicts an Ab that binds to an nsEV surface marker tetraspanin protein such as CD63) onto Dynabeads Epoxy and also has flexibility in choosing the Ab used to detect the nsEV surface protein being quantified. A PE-conjugated anti-nsEV surface protein Ab may be used as an alternative to the primary biotinylated Ab/secondary PE-conjugated streptavidin labeling approach shown in the figure

2. The concentration of anti-nsEV surface protein Ab providing an optimal balance between fluorescence signal dynamic range and nonspecific Ab binding (*see* **Note 10**) to Dynabeads-nsEV complexes must be determined empirically. The author has obtained satisfactory results with both biotin- and phycoery-thrin (PE)-conjugated anti-nsEV surface protein Abs incubated with Dynabeads-nsEV complexes at a concentration of 1 μg/mL.

3. After completing **step 9** in Subheading 3.2 above, resuspend Dynabeads in 500 μL of room temperature PBSL and the empirically determined concentration of primary anti-nsEV surface protein Ab. Incubations carried out using PE-conjugated anti-nsEV surface protein Abs should be performed in the dark to prevent photobleaching of the PE fluorophores. Alternatively, PE fluorophores can be protected from light by covering the lab rotator's tube holder with aluminum foil.

4. Allow Dynabeads-nsEV complex labeling to proceed on a lab rotator (*see* **Note 5**) for 2 h at room temperature.

5. Perform two 1-min wash steps using the DynaMag and bench-top minifuge as described in **step 7** of Subheading 3.2. Perform the first wash with PBS containing PBSW and the second wash with PBSA.

6. For Dynabeads-nsEV complexes that have been labeled with PE-conjugated anti-nsEV surface protein Abs proceed to **step 9** in Subheading 3.3.

7. For Dynabeads-nsEV complexes that have been labeled with biotinylated anti-nsEV surface protein Abs perform secondary labeling with PE-conjugated streptavidin by resuspending

Dynabeads-nsEV complexes in 500 μL of PBSL containing 10 μg/mL PE-conjugated streptavidin and rotating, with protection from light to prevent photobleaching, on a lab rotator for 30 min.

8. After the 30-min secondary labeling incubation is complete, perform a single wash using PBSW.

9. Resuspend washed Dynabeads-nsEV complexes in 700 μL of PBS that does not contain BSA for flow cytometric analysis. Resuspended Dynabeads-nsEV complexes should be protected from light during the interval between resuspension and loading onto the flow cytometer to prevent PE photobleaching. Representative flow cytometry assay results obtained using the procedures described here in Subheading 3.3 appear in Figs. 3 and 4.

3.4 Magnetic Particle ELISA Colorimetric Quantification of Surface Proteins Presented by Magnetic Particle-Bound nsEVs

1. The magnetic particle ELISA described below is an attractive alternative to flow cytometry for cases in which one desires increased nsEV surface protein detection sensitivity or has limited access to flow cytometry apparatuses. As is the case for flow cytometric quantification of nsEV surface proteins present on Dynabeads-bound nsEVs, quantification of nsEV surface proteins is achieved by measuring binding of anti-nsEV surface

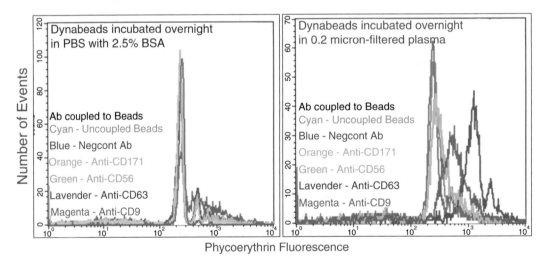

Fig. 3 Flow cytometry histograms showing ability to specifically enrich nsEVs from plasma using Dynabeads Epoxy coupled with various anti-nsEV surface protein Abs. After incubation in plasma or PBS with 2.5% (w/v), BSA as a negative control Dynabeads were labeled with PE-conjugated anti-CD9 Ab. *Y*-axis denotes number of Dynabeads events counted by flow cytometer, *X*-axis denotes phycoerythrin (PE) fluorescence signals. Legends in lower left corner of histograms denote the Abs that have been coupled to Dynabeads Epoxy surfaces. Left panel histogram corresponds to analysis of Dynabeads incubated with PBS/2.5% BSA rather than plasma; these histograms show that PE-conjugated anti-CD9 Ab has low propensity to nonspecifically bind Ab-coupled Dynabeads. CD56 and CD171 are neuronal nsEV surface marker proteins. Dynabeads coupled with anti-CD56 or anti-CD171 Abs IP far fewer plasma nsEVs than Dynabeads coupled with Abs binding the respective generic nsEV surface marker tetraspanins CD9 and CD63. This outcome is expected based on neuron-derived nsEVs accounting for a relatively small fraction of the total plasma nsEV population [4]

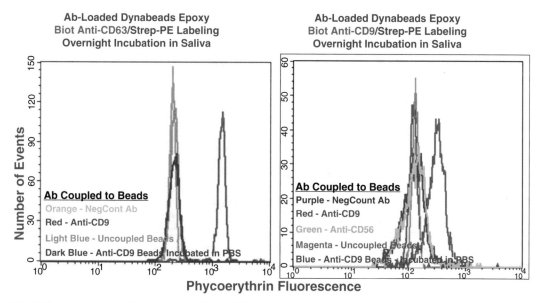

Fig. 4 Flow cytometry histograms showing ability to specifically enrich nsEVs from saliva using Dynabeads coupled with anti-CD9 Abs. After incubation of Ab-coupled Dynabeads in saliva, Ab-loaded Dynabeads-nsEV complexes were labeled with PE-conjugated anti-CD63 (*left panel*) or anti-CD9 (*right panel*) Ab for flow cytometric analysis. Y-axis denotes number of Dynabeads events counted by flow cytometer. X-axis denotes anti-nsEV tetraspanin marker PE-conjugated Ab fluorescence. Legends in lower left corner of histograms denote Abs coupled to Dynabeads. Ab-coupled Dynabeads were incubated with both saliva and PBS with 2.5% BSA with the latter incubation serving as a negative control for nonspecific binding of PE-conjugated anti-CD9 Ab to Dynabeads surfaces. Phosphate-citrate buffer, pH 5.0, was used for high stringency washing during nsEV IP

protein Abs to surface proteins presented by Dynabeads-bound nsEVs that have been IPed using the procedure of Subheading 3.2 (Fig. 5).

The magnetic particle ELISA's increased nsEV surface protein detection sensitivity relative to the flow cytometric assay of Subheading 3.3 is enabled by the ELISA's compatibility with utilization of horseradish peroxidase (HRP)-conjugated streptavidin as a secondary label after primary labeling of Dynabeads-nsEV complexes with biotinylated anti-nsEV surface protein Ab. HRP-conjugated streptavidin enables increased sensitivity by facilitating enzyme-mediated signal amplification; each HRP molecule can catalyze multiple conversions of a colorless colorimetric substrate, where satisfactory results have been obtained using a commercially available 3,3′,5,5′-Tetramethylbenzidine (TMB) solution, into a product molecule that strongly absorbs light at a specific wavelength, e.g., 450 nm for TMB, in the visible spectrum and is thus easily quantified using a standard 96-well platereader.

In contrast to magnetic particle ELISA quantification of nsEV surface proteins, the flow cytometric quantification

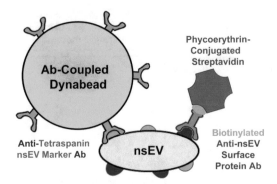

Fig. 5 Magnetic particle ELISA surface protein quantification schematic. The researcher is free to couple any Ab of interest (figure depicts an Ab that binds to an nsEV surface marker tetraspanin protein such as CD63) onto Dynabeads Epoxy and also has flexibility in choosing the Ab used to detect the nsEV surface protein being quantified. Magnetic particle ELISA quantification of nsEV surface protein abundance requires use of a biotinylated anti-nsEV surface protein primary Ab and HRP-conjugated streptavidin as a secondary labeling agent

method of Subheading 3.2 does not enable one to leverage enzyme-mediated signal amplification to enhance detection sensitivity. This inability arises from each Dynabeads-nsEV complex being deposited in the cytometer's waste reservoir after a single pass through the beam emitted by the flow cytometer's excitation laser; each Dynabeads-nsEV complex bound fluorophore has only one opportunity to contribute to the increase in fluorescence signal observed for anti-nsEV surface protein Ab-bound Dynabeads-nsEV complexes relative to the background fluorescence observed for Dynabeads-nsEV complexes that are not bound by anti-nsEV surface protein Abs.

2. The concentration of anti-nsEV surface protein Ab providing an optimal balance between fluorescence signal dynamic range and nonspecific Ab binding (*see* **Note 10**) to Dynabeads-nsEV complexes must be determined empirically. The author has obtained satisfactory results by using biotinylated anti-nsEV surface protein Abs incubated with Dynabeads-nsEV complexes at a concentration of 1 µg/mL.

3. After completing **step 9** in Subheading 3.2 above, resuspend Dynabeads in **500** µL of room temperature PBSL and the empirically determined concentration of biotinylated anti-nsEV surface protein Ab.

4. Allow Dynabeads-nsEV complex labeling to proceed on a lab rotator (*see* **Note 5**) for 2 h at room temperature.

5. Perform three 1-min wash steps using the DynaMag and benchtop minifuge as described in **step 7** of Subheading 3.2. Perform the first wash with PBSW and carry out the second and third washes using PBSA. After the first step and resuspen-

sion in PBSA transfer, Dynabeads-nsEV complexes to a new microfuge tube to minimize carryover of unbound biotinylated antibody. Such carryover can increase background signals during colorimetric quantification of nsEV surface marker proteins as described below in **steps 8–11**.

6. Perform secondary labeling of Dynabeads-nsEV complexes by resuspending in 500 μL of PBSL containing 0.5 μg/mL HRP-conjugated streptavidin and rotating on a lab rotator for 30 min.

7. After the 30-min secondary labeling incubation is complete execute the washing and microfuge tube transfer steps as described in **step 5** of Subheading 3.4. Extreme care should be taken to completely remove all wash buffer from the microfuge tubes after the final wash.

8. Prepare Dynabeads-nsEV complexes for colorimetric quantification of nsEV surface proteins by resuspending the complexes in 65 μL of PBS. Perform duplicate nsEV surface protein measurements for each biofluid specimen from which nsEVs were IPed. For each measurement, dilute 20 μL of the resuspended Dynabeads-nsEV complexes with 20 μL of PBS in a fresh microfuge tube and then add 100 μL of Ultra TMB ELISA substrate to each of these tubes (*see* **Notes 11** and **12**). Vortex tubes for a few seconds at an intermediate speed 2–4 times at intervals throughout the 15-min substrate development period during which the colorless substrate molecule is converted by HRP into a blue-colored product molecule (*see* **Note 13**). After 15 min of substrate development, add 140 μL of 2 N sulfuric acid to each microfuge tube to halt the color development. In addition to halting HRP-catalyzed substrate conversion, this acidification step will cause the blue product molecule to change color and cause the aqueous solution in which the product conversion reaction has occurred to become yellow.

9. Centrifuge the microfuge tubes containing both the yellow reaction solution and the magnetic particle-nsEV complexes at 13,000 rcf for 2 min to pellet the magnetic particles and transfer 200 μL of each supernatant to one well of a transparent flatbottom 96-well plate.

10. Measure absorbances, which are proportional to the amount of TMB substrate that has been converted by HRP, for each well at 450 nm using a microplate reader. Subtract absorbance values (typically around 0.05 absorbance units) for a blank well containing 200 μL of a 2.5:1 (v/v) mixture of ELISA substrate and PBS from the absorbance values for each nsEV IP substrate conversion reaction supernatant.

11. Analyze absorbance data to determine the relative amounts of the nsEV surface protein of interest that has been isolated in each IP. Representative magnetic particle ELISA results

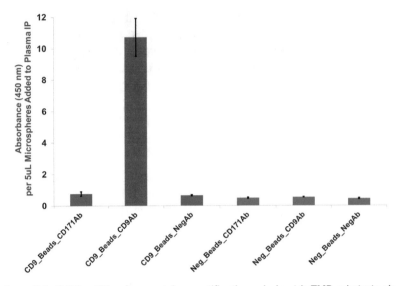

Fig. 6 Magnetic particle ELISA nsEV surface protein quantification colorimetric TMB substrate absorbance data for various Ab-coupled Dynabeads incubated overnight with plasma. The first Abs denoted by the *X*-axis labels are the Abs coupled onto Dynabeads Epoxy for use in nsEV IP from plasma. The second Abs denoted by the *X*-axis labels are the biotinylated Abs used for nsEV surface protein quantification. Dynabeads-nsEV complex secondary labeling was performed with HRP-conjugated streptavidin. CD171 is a neuronal nsEV surface protein marker. As neuron-derived nsEVs account for a relatively small fraction of the total plasma nsEV population [4] it is unsurprising that absorbances above background are not observed for use of biotinylated anti-CD171 Ab to quantify CD171 on the surfaces of plasma nsEVs IPed using anti-CD9 Ab-coupled Dynabeads. Use of biotinylated anti-CD171 detection Ab to quantify CD171 presented by anti-CD171 Ab-coupled Dynabeads after incubation with plasma and high stringency washing results in a robust absorbance signal similar to that of the anti-CD9/anti-CD9-coupled Ab/detection Ab pairing (*red bar*) appearing in the figure (CD171/CD171 data not shown). Error bars denote standard deviations for four replicates

obtained using the procedures described here in Subheading 3.4 appear in Fig. 6.

3.5 Quantification of Magnetic Particle-Immunoprecipitated nsEV Protein Constituents

1. Methods that the author has employed for shotgun proteomic profiling of Dynabeads-IPed nsEVs are described at length elsewhere [21].

2. Individual or small sets of both intravesicular and surface nsEV proteins can be quantified via ELISA [4–8] or other fluorescent [16, 26] immunoassays. A wide range of nsEV lysis and membrane protein extraction methods, the majority of which utilize either commercial cell lysis reagents or detergent-containing buffers, have been described in the literature [4–8]. In applying these lysis and protein extraction methods, one begins by resuspending the washed Dynabeads-nsEV complexes output from **step 9** in Subheading 3.2 above in appropriate lysis

buffer (*see* **Note 14**) and then proceeds to execute the ELISA or fluorescent immunoassay procedural steps, possibly with modifications and/or added steps to account for the presence of Dynabeads, described in the journal article or manufacturer's product literature being followed.

3.6 Quantification of Magnetic Particle-Immunoprecipitated Nucleic Acid Constituents

1. The nsEV IP method of Subheading 3.1 has been used as a lead-in to successful RT-PCR amplification of nsEV miRNAs from total RNA that was extracted from IPed nsEVs. The procedures discussed here in Subheading 3.6 could also be used, where scaleup and/or modification of the IP procedure and nucleic acid isolation protocol may be required, to enable quantification of individual nsEV messenger RNAs (mRNAs) or other nsEV nucleic acid species such as double-stranded DNA [27]. Additionally, the IP methods of Subheading 3.1 could be used to isolate nsEV nucleic acids for use in commercial kit-based construction of nsEV nucleic acid libraries that are compatible with omics level nsEV nucleic acid profiling via NGS.

2. Execution of the miRNeasy Micro Kit manufacturer's protocol for 50 μL scale extraction of total nsEV RNA has enabled extraction of miRNA from Dynabeads-nsEV complexes. When specimen volumes permit, the author recommends performing two duplicate nsEV IPs, e.g., two identical 1.2 mL scale plasma nsEV IPs, for each 50 μL scale extraction when miRNA is being isolated for downstream qRT-PCR quantification of individual nsEV miRNAs; this IP scaleup increases post-extraction miRNA yield (*see* **Note 15**). The first step of the RNA extraction procedure should be modified such that Dynabeads-nsEV complexes output from **step 9** in Subheading 3.2 above, absent any resuspension buffer, are substituted for the 50 μL RNA-containing liquid sample described in the manufacturer's instructions.

3. Although other RNA quantification methods may be used, satisfactory results have been obtained with the RiboGreen assay kit. Pooling Dynabeads-nsEV complexes obtained from duplicate nsEV IPs allows single-digit nanogram or greater amounts, as quantified using the RiboGreen assay, of total RNA to be extracted from IPed nsEVs.

4. Use extracted nsEV nucleic acids in downstream applications, such as qRT-PCR determination of individual miRNAs, as desired. Representative miRNA threshold cycle (C_t) determination plots generated by qRT-PCR analysis of total nsEV RNA isolated using the methods described here in Subheading 3.6 appear in Fig. 7.

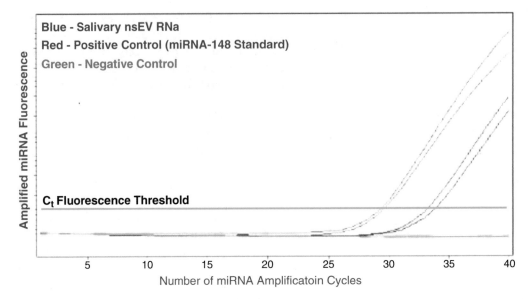

Fig. 7 qRT-PCR amplification signal intensity plot for miRNA-148, which is enriched in salivary nsEVs [28, 29], contained within RNA extracted from salivary nsEVs IPed using the Dynabeads CD81 Exosome Isolation product and for respective positive and negative control miRNA amplifications. Y-axis denotes fluorescence intensity (proportional to amount of miRNA). X-axis denotes number of reaction cycles required for fluorescence to exceed chosen threshold (one arbitrary fluorescence unit) for these assays. *Blue lines*: salivary nsEV RNA fluorescence for duplicate reactions. *Red lines*: miRNA standard (positive control) fluorescence. *Green lines*: negative control reactions using manufacturer's negative control RNA as template. Respective C_t values for salivary nsEV RNA and miRNA-148 standard duplicate reactions: 28.6 cycles, 28.7 cycles and 32.1 cycles, 32.8 cycles

4 Notes

1. It is important to note that regardless of what magnetic particles are used the nsEV-binding Abs must be covalently coupled to particles. Noncovalently coupled Abs, e.g., biotinylated Abs bound to streptavidin-coupled magnetic particles, may dissociate from magnetic particles during nsEV protein or nucleic acid extraction steps and could interfere with downstream analyses. Such Ab dissociation is particularly problematic in the context of mass spectrometric proteomic analysis as dissociated Abs lead to contamination of the peptide ion spectra.

2. Washes following the low pH wash are performed using Buffer E1 from the Dynabeads Antibody Coupling kit; 0.025% (v/v) Tween-20 should be added to Buffer E1 before use.

3. Dynabeads M-270 Epoxy are packaged dry by the manufacturer and have a density of ~6.7 × 10⁷ particles/mg. The author has typically resuspended Ab-coupled Dynabeads at a concentration of 10 mg/mL, or ~6.8 × 10⁸ particles/mL, in Buffer E1 with 0.025% Tween-20 after Ab coupling and washing. Ab-coupled Dynabeads Epoxy can be stored for up to 6 weeks at 4 °C following coupling with no apparent loss of

nsEV-binding capacity. Although the author has not added azide to Ab-coupled Dynabeads prior to storage, care has been taken to avoid nonchalant handling procedures that could lead to microbial contamination of Ab-coupled Dynabeads stocks.

4. The recommended 5 μL aliquot of Ab-coupled Dynabeads for plasma nsEV IP, which results in a greater number of Dynabeads per unit volume plasma than the aliquots of preloaded anti CD9, CD63, and CD81 Dynabeads specified in **step 2** of Subheading 3.2, is utilized to reduce the likelihood of both pipetting inaccurate liquid volumes and drawing aliquots of Dynabeads that are not uniformly suspended in the storage buffer; the probability of both of these phenomena increases with decreasing transfer volume. If one desires to make comparisons of anti-tissue type marker Ab-coupled and CD9, CD63, or CD81 Dynabeads using equal numbers of magnetic particles in each IP one should dilute Ab-coupled Dynabeads Epoxy in PBS so that transfer volumes remain at or above 5 μL. The lower cost of Ab-coupled Dynabeads Epoxy on a per magnetic particle basis relative to the CD9, CD63, and CD81 Dynabeads Exosome Isolation reagents has motivated the author's use of fewer Dynabeads in IP performed with the latter three products.

5. To minimize foaming during incubation of anti-nsEV surface protein Abs with Dynabeads, one may reposition the lab rotator's tube holding rack so that microfuge tubes rotate side-over-side rather than head-over-head. The author has observed that appreciable foaming can occur when 1.5 mL microfuge tubes containing less than 700–800 μL of liquid are rotated head-over-head for intervals of greater than approximately 15 min. The likelihood of observing such foaming is particularly acute when the liquid in the tubes being rotated is protein rich, e.g., biofluid specimens or buffers containing BSA concentrations at or above approximately 0.1%.

6. For biofluids that contain lower nsEV concentrations than plasma and serum, e.g., saliva, it has been observed that washing in pH 3 buffer removes nsEVs from Dynabeads to a degree that precludes nsEV detection via flow cytometry or magnetic particle ELISA. Carrying out the low pH washes in 25 mM phosphate-citrate buffer, pH 5.0 provides a desirable balance between satisfactory nsEV capture and low nonspecific adsorption of nsEVs to Dynabeads surfaces as determined via flow cytometric analysis of Dynabeads after nsEV IP (Fig. 4).

7. Adsorption of BSA to plasticware surfaces, nsEVs, and Dynabeads can result in contamination of the peptide ion spectra obtained during tandem mass spectrometric profiling of nsEV proteomes [21]. This albumin contamination issue can

be mitigated by employing modified Dynabeads wash conditions that employ BSA-free buffers [21].

8. The strength of the multivalent interaction between the anti-nsEV Abs coupled to Dynabeads surfaces and the nsEVs that remain bound to Dynabeads after washing has been completed precludes subsequent analysis of IPed nsEVs using electron microscopy or NanoSight analysis. Efforts to elute detectable numbers of intact nsEVs from Dynabeads surfaces using both commercial nsEV elution buffers and nsEV elution buffers described in publications in which nsEV IP procedures that do not feature stringent wash conditions [4–8] were employed have been unsuccessful.

9. Regardless of whether biotinylated anti-nsEV surface protein Abs in conjunction with fluorescent streptavidin secondary labeling or fluorescent anti-nsEV surface protein Abs are used for flow cytometric nsEV surface marker protein quantification phycoerythrin (PE) should be employed as the detection fluorophore whenever possible. The author has observed that use of PE-conjugated primary Abs and PE-conjugated streptavidin leads to markedly increased flow cytometry fluorescence signals relative to Abs and streptavidin conjugated with either fluorescein isothiocyanate (FITC) or Alexa dyes.

Although it is reasonable to anticipate that biotinylated primary Ab labeling followed by secondary labeling with PE-conjugated streptavidin would lead to more robust fluorescence signals than single-step labeling with PE-conjugated primary anti-nsEV surface protein Abs similar fluorescence signal dynamic ranges have typically been observed regardless of whether single-step or two-step fluorescent labeling of Dynabeads-nsEV complexes is performed. The limited breadth of commercially available PE primary Ab conjugates and relative paucity of publications describing successful use of PE Ab conjugation kits provides motivation for performing two-step labeling with biotinylated Abs as the primary detection agent; primary Abs specific for a wide range of nsEV surface proteins are commercially available and methods for Ab biotinylation using N-hydroxsuccinimidyl (NHS) biotin esters, such as ThermoFisher Scientific EZ-Link Sulfo-NHS-LC-sulfobiotin, are well established and have been described in hundreds of publications.

10. Background fluorescence signals can arise from either specific binding of anti-nsEV surface protein Abs to nsEVs that are nonspecifically adsorbed on Dynabeads surfaces or nonspecific binding of anti-nsEV surface protein Abs to the surfaces of Dynabeads-nsEV complexes. Although the number of nsEVs nonspecifically adsorbed on Dynabeads surfaces is expected to be extremely small when stringent low pH washing is applied

during IP, one may wish to perform flow cytometry experiments with negative control Ab-coupled Dynabeads to verify the specificity of nsEV IP by anti-nsEV surface protein-coupled Dynabeads.

Negative control Ab-coupled Dynabeads can be prepared using the method described in **step 2** of Subheading 3.2 to covalently link negative control isotype-matched Abs to Dynabeads Epoxy surfaces. The author is not aware of a Dynabeads product that serves as an appropriate control for nonspecific nsEV adsorption on Ab-coupled Dynabeads surfaces. Nonspecific binding of anti-nsEV surface protein Abs to the surfaces of Dynabeads used for nsEV IP can be assessed by incubating Dynabeads-nsEV complexes with biotinylated or PE-conjugated Abs possessing isotypes matching the isotypes of the PE- or biotin-conjugated Abs used for nsEV surface protein quantification.

11. To prevent HRP contamination of the TMB substrate solution, remove an aliquot of the required amount of substrate solution from the bottle, which should be stored at 4 °C, prior to addition to the resuspended Dynabeads-nsEV complexes. Allow the aliquot of substrate solution to equilibrate to room temperature prior to adding to the resuspended Dynabeads; allowing the HRP-catalyzed TMB substrate conversion to occur at room temperature enhances color development relative to carrying out the conversion using cold substrate solution. The substrate solution is light sensitive and should be protected from light during the room temperature equilibration interval. Removal of the substrate solution aliquot from the stock bottle stored at 4 °C should be timed such that the substrate solution is equilibrated to room temperature and ready to add to Dynabeads-nsEV complexes immediately after resuspension of the Dynabeads in PBS.

12. Extreme care should be taken to prevent pipette tips from contacting the liquid in the 96-well plate during the addition of TMB substrate solution. Even a single μL of liquid carryover into the master tube containing the TMB solution can result in HRP contamination and unintended conversion of substrate within the master tube. Using a fresh pipette tip for each substrate solution draw and addition to the 96-well plate is a tractable avenue for preventing such contamination.

13. Prevent light-induced degradation of the TMB substrate by placing microfuge tubes in a drawer or under aluminum foil during the time periods between each interval of vortexing.

14. Due to the potential for lysis reagent components to interfere with ELISA and/or immunoassay quantification of nsEV proteins, one must often empirically assess whether a particular

nsEV lysis method is compatible with the researcher's preferred downstream nsEV protein quantification assay(s).

15. Dynabeads-nsEV complexes obtained from duplicate IPs should be pooled prior to executing the first step of the manufacturer's RNA extraction protocol.

References

1. Cocucci E, Meldolesi J (2015) Ectosomes and exosomes: shedding the confusion between extracellular vesicles. Trends Cell Biol 25:364–372

2. Yoshioka Y et al (2014) Ultra-sensitive liquid biopsy of circulating extracellular vesicles using ExoScreen. Nat Commun 5:3591

3. He M, Crow J, Roth M, Zeng Y, Godwin AK (2014) Integrated immunoisolation and protein analysis of circulating exosomes using microfluidic technology. Lab Chip 14:3773–3780

4. Fiandaca MS, Kapogiannis D, Mapstone M, Boxer A, Eitan E, Schwartz JB, Abner EL, Petersen RC, Federoff HJ, Miller BL, Goetzl EJ (2015) Identification of preclinical Alzheimer's disease by a profile of pathogenic proteins in neurally derived blood exosomes: a case-control study. Alzheimers Dement 11:600–607

5. Goetzl EJ, Boxer A, Schwartz JB, Abner EL, Petersen RC, Miller BL, Kapogiannis D (2015) Altered lysosomal proteins in neural-derived plasma exosomes in preclinical Alzheimer disease. Neurology 85(1):40–47

6. Goetzl EJ, Boxer A, Schwartz JB, Abner EL, Petersen RC, Miller BL, Carlson OD, Mustapic M, Kapogiannis D (2015) Low neural exosomal levels of cellular survival factors in Alzheimer's disease. Ann Clin Transl Neurol 2:769–773

7. Kapogiannis D, Boxer A, Schwartz JB, Abner EL, Biragyn A, Masharani U, Frassetto L, Petersen RC, Miller BL, Goetzl EJ (2015) Dysfunctionally phosphorylated type 1 insulin receptor substrate in neural-derived blood exosomes of preclinical Alzheimer's disease. FASEB J 29(2):589–596

8. Shi M, Liu C, Cook TJ, Bullock KM, Zhao Y, Ginghina C, Li Y, Aro P, Dator R, He C, Hipp MJ, Zabetian CP, Peskind ER, Hu SC, Quinn JF, Galasko DR, Banks WA, Zhang J (2014) Plasma exosomal α-synuclein is likely CNS-derived and increased in Parkinson's disease. Acta Neuropathol 128:639–650

9. Schey K, Luther J, Rose K (2015) Proteomics characterization of exosome cargo. Methods 87:75–82

10. Laurent LC, Abdel-Mageed AB, Adelson PD, Arango J, Balaj L, Breakefield X, Carlson E, Carter BS, Majem B, Chen CC, Cocucci E, Danielson K, Courtright A, Das S, Abd Elmageed ZY, Enderle D, Ezrin A, Ferrer M, Freedman J, Galas D, Gandhi R, Huentelman MJ, Van Keuren-Jensen K, Kalani Y, Kim Y, Krichevsky AM, Lai C, Lal-Nag M, Laurent CD, Leonardo T, Li F, Malenica I, Mondal D, Nejad P, Patel T, Raffai RL, Rubio R, Skog J, Spetzler R, Sun J, Tanriverdi K, Vickers K, Wang L, Wang Y, Wei Z, Weiner HL, Wong D, Yan IK, Yeri A, Gould S (2015) Meeting report: discussions and preliminary findings on extracellular RNA measurement methods from laboratories in the NIH Extracellular RNA Communication Consortium. J Extracell Vesicles 4:26533

11. Giallombardo M, Chacártegui Borrás J, Castiglia M, Van Der Steen N, Mertens I, Pauwels P, Peeters M, Rolfo C (2016) Exosomal miRNA analysis in non-small cell lung cancer (NSCLC) patients' plasma through qPCR: a feasible liquid biopsy tool. J Vis Exp (111)

12. Caradec J, Kharmate G, Hosseini-Beheshti E, Adomat H, Gleave M, Guns E (2014) Reproducibility and efficiency of serum-derived exosome extraction methods. Clin Biochem 47:1286–1292

13. Kanninen KM, Bister N, Koistinaho J, Malm T (2015) Exosomes as new diagnostic tools in CNS diseases. Biochim Biophys Acta S09:292–296

14. Webber J, Clayton A (2013) How pure are your vesicles? J Extracell Vesicles 10:2. https://doi.org/10.3402/jev.v2i0.19861

15. Xie H, Griffin TJ (2006) Trade-off between high sensitivity and increased potential for false positive peptide sequence matches using a two-dimensional linear ion trap for tandem mass spectrometry-based proteomics. J Proteome Res 5(4):1003–1009

16. Franquesa M, Hoogduijn MJ, Ripoll E, Luk F, Salih M, Betjes MG, Torras J, Baan CC, Grinyó JM, Merino AM (2014) Update on controls for isolation and quantification methodology

of extracellular vesicles derived from adipose tissue mesenchymal stem cells. Front Immunol 5:525

17. Elshimali YI, Khaddour H, Sarkissyan M, Wu Y, Vadgama JV (2013) The clinical utilization of circulating cell free DNA (CCFDNA) in blood of cancer patients. Int J Mol Sci 14(9):18925–18958

18. Rudnick SI, Adams GP (2007) Affinity and avidity in antibody-based tumor targeting. Cancer Biother Radiopharm 24:155–161

19. Perez-Gonzalez R, Gauthier SA, Kumar A, Levy E (2012) The exosome secretory pathway transports amyloid precursor protein carboxyl-terminal fragments from the cell into the brain extracellular space. J Biol Chem 287:43108–43115

20. Heinzelman P, Bilousova T, Campagna J, John V (2016) Nanoscale extracellular vesicle analysis in Alzheimer's disease diagnosis and therapy. Int J Alzheimers Dis 2016:8053139

21. Heinzelman P, Powers D, Wohlschlegel J, John V (2017). Shotgun proteomic profiling of bloodborne nanoscale extracellular vesicles. Book chapter in press at Methods in Biobanking

22. Shi M, Kovac A, Korff A, Cook TJ, Ginghina C, Bullock KM, Yang L, Stewart T, Zheng D, Aro P, Atik A, Kerr KF, Zabetian CP, Peskind ER, Hu SC, Quinn JF, Galasko DR, Montine TJ, Banks WA, Zhang J (2016) CNS tau efflux via exosomes is likely increased in Parkinson's disease but not in Alzheimer's disease. Alzheimers Dement 12:1125–1131

23. Crossland R, Norden J, Bibby L, Davis J, Dickinson A (2016) Evaluation of optimal extracellular vesicle small RNA isolation and qRT-PCR normalisation for serum and urine. J Immunol Methods 429:39–49

24. Momen-Heravi F, Balaj L, Alian S, Trachtenberg AJ, Hochberg FH, Skog J, Kuo WP (2012) Impact of biofluid viscosity on size and sedimentation efficiency of the isolated microvesicles. Front Physiol 3:162

25. Chen WW, Balaj L, Liau LM, Samuels ML, Kotsopoulos SK, Maguire CA, Loguidice L, Soto H, Garrett M, Zhu LD, Sivaraman S, Chen C, Wong ET, Carter BS, Hochberg FH, Breakefield XO, Skog J (2013) BEAMing and droplet digital PCR analysis of mutant IDH1 mRNA in glioma patient serum and cerebrospinal fluid extracellular vesicles. Mol Ther Nucleic Acids 2:e109

26. Stern RA, Tripodis Y, Baugh CM, Fritts NG, Martin BM, Chaisson C, Cantu RC, Joyce JA, Shah S, Ikezu T, Zhang J, Gercel-Taylor C, Taylor DD (2016) Preliminary study of plasma exosomal tau as a potential biomarker for chronic traumatic encephalopathy. J Alzheimers Dis 51:1099–1109

27. Thakur BK, Zhang H, Becker A, Matei I, Huang Y, Costa-Silva B, Zheng Y, Hoshino A, Brazier H, Xiang J, Williams C, Rodriguez-Barrueco R, Silva JM, Zhang W, Hearn S, Elemento O, Paknejad N, Manova-Todorova K, Welte K, Bromberg J, Peinado H, Lyden D (2014) Double-stranded DNA in exosomes: a novel biomarker in cancer detection. Cell Res 24:766–769

28. Matse JH, Yoshizawa J, Wang X, Elashoff D, Bolscher JG, Leemans CR, Pegtel MD, Wong DT, Bloemena E (2015) Human salivary micro-RNA in patients with parotid salivary gland neoplasms. PLoS One 10(11):e0142264

29. Matse JH, Yoshizawa J, Wang X, Elashoff D, Bolscher JG, Veerman EC, Bloemena E, Wong DT (2013) Discovery and prevalidation of salivary extracellular microRNA biomarkers panel for the noninvasive detection of benign and malignant parotid gland tumors. Clin Cancer Res 19:3032–3038

Chapter 9

Enrichment of Extracellular Vesicle Subpopulations Via Affinity Chromatography

Michelle E. Hung, Stephen B. Lenzini, Devin M. Stranford, and Joshua N. Leonard

Abstract

Extracellular vesicles (EVs) are secreted nanoscale particles that transfer biomolecular cargo between cells in multicellular organisms. EVs play a variety of roles in intercellular communication and are being explored as potential vehicles for delivery of therapeutic biomolecules. However, EVs are highly heterogeneous in composition and biogenesis route, and this poses substantial challenges for understanding the role of EVs in biology and for harnessing these mechanisms for therapeutic applications, for which purifying therapeutic EVs from mixed EV populations may be necessary. Currently, technologies for isolating EV subsets are limited by overlapping physical properties among EV subsets. To meet this need, here we report an affinity chromatography-based method for enriching a specific EV subset from a heterogeneous EV starting population. By displaying an affinity tagged protein (tag-protein) on the EV surface, tagged EVs may be specifically isolated using simple affinity chromatography. Moreover, recovered EVs are enriched in the tag-protein relative to the starting population of EVs and relative to EVs purified from cell culture supernatant by standard differential centrifugation. Furthermore, chromatographically enriched EVs confer enhanced delivery of a cargo protein to recipient cells (via enhancing the amount of cargo protein per EV) relative to EVs isolated by centrifugation. Altogether, affinity chromatographic enrichment of EV subsets is a viable and facile strategy for investigating EV biology and for harnessing EVs for therapeutic applications.

Key words Chromatography, Exosome, Microvesicle, Purification, Vesicle

1 Introduction

Extracellular vesicles (EVs) are secreted nanoscale particles that mediate intercellular communication via the exchange of biomolecules [1, 2]. EVs encapsulate RNA, proteins, and other membrane-associated and cytoplasmic species, all of which can be transferred to recipient cells via EV uptake and membrane fusion. EV-mediated communication plays a role in many physiological processes, including stem cell maintenance, regulation of immune responses, and tissue repair after injury as well as pathological processes including viral transfer, enhancing tumor invasion and angiogenesis, and

Tushar Patel (ed.), *Extracellular RNA: Methods and Protocols*, Methods in Molecular Biology, vol. 1740,
https://doi.org/10.1007/978-1-4939-7652-2_9, © Springer Science+Business Media, LLC 2018

transfer of toxic proteins in neurodegenerative disorders. EVs secreted from different cell types can vary significantly in lipid, protein, and RNA content, and these variations enable the many different biological roles played by EVs from different sources. Moreover, even EVs secreted from a single cell type comprise a heterogeneous population [3, 4]. EVs include apoptotic bodies (micron-sized particles secreted from cells undergoing apoptosis), microvesicles (nanoscale particles that bud from the cell surface), and exosomes (nanoscale particles that derive from invagination of endosomal membranes). Each of these vesicle subpopulations has distinct RNA, protein, and lipid contents and plays a distinct role in intercellular communication. Even within these EV categories, subpopulations with different properties exist. For example, when H5V endothelial cell-derived exosomes were separated into subsets by density gradient centrifugation, exposure of H5V recipient cells to different exosome subsets induced distinct patterns of gene expression [5]. While EV heterogeneity is well documented, methods for studying specific EV subsets are limited.

Isolating homogeneous (or less heterogeneous) populations of vesicles is challenging and time-consuming. One challenge is that microvesicles and exosomes often overlap in size and density such that differential centrifugation methods used to purify vesicles from cell culture supernatant often yield mixtures of different types of EVs [3]. Sucrose gradient centrifugation can be used to separate microvesicles and exosomes, but this method is time-consuming and may require further downstream purification to remove the sucrose if EVs are to be delivered to cells. Moreover, density-based separation may still result in the isolation of heterogeneous vesicle populations in terms of protein or RNA content. To dissect the biology of different EV subpopulations, methods for isolating specific EV subpopulations are needed.

Affinity-based purification of EVs is a promising method for isolating EV subsets, but new approaches are needed for many applications. Methods for isolation of exosomes, which are often defined by the presence of CD63 in the membrane, have been developed by using magnetic beads conjugated to an anti-CD63 antibody [6]. Similar approaches targeting other exosome membrane proteins including MHCII (for dendritic cell-derived EVs), the transferrin receptor, and colon cancer antigen A33 [7] have been used for immunoisolation of exosomes. However, each of these methods is applicable only to analytical applications, in which elution of intact EVs from the capture beads is not required or has not been evaluated. In this chapter, we report a method for EV isolation by affinity chromatography, which enables enrichment of a specific subset of intact EVs (Fig. 1). The method presented here can conceivably be generalized to isolate EV subsets displaying any protein of interest.

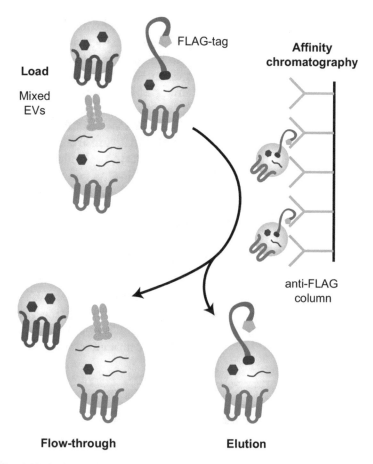

Fig. 1 Method overview: recovery of EVs via affinity chromatography. This cartoon summarizes the strategy for isolating EVs by affinity chromatography. A heterogeneous population of EVs is loaded on an anti-FLAG affinity column, EVs displaying FLAG peptide are retained on the column while other EVs flow through the column, and upon elution with FLAG peptide, an enriched population of FLAG-positive EVs is recovered

2 Materials

2.1 Cell Culture

1. 5% CO_2 tissue culture incubator, humidified, with temperature set at 37 °C.

2. 15 cm tissue culture plates.

3. EV-producing cells of interest; in this chapter, HEK293FT cells (Thermo-Fisher Scientific) were used.

4. EV-depleted growth medium for cells (**item 3**). FBS is a source of EVs, so medium must be depleted of EVs either by use of EV-depleted FBS (available commercially) or by removal of EVs from medium by ultracentrifugation. If ultracentrifugation is chosen, additional materials required include an ultra-

centrifuge, ultracentrifuge rotor, and ultracentrifuge tubes compatible with EV isolation by ultracentrifugation (described in greater detail elsewhere [6]). Here, EV-depleted medium was generated by pelleting FBS-derived EVs from DMEM containing 20% FBS by ultracentrifugation at 120,094 × g in an Optima XP ultracentrifuge (Beckman Coulter) with the SW41Ti rotor for 135 min at 4 °C. The cleared supernatant was mixed with serum-free supplemented Dulbecco's Modified Eagle's Medium (1% Penicillin Streptomycin, 4 mM L-glutamine) to achieve a final concentration of 10% FBS in "EV-depleted medium." Extending this ultracentrifugation step may further remove residual FBS-derived EVs [6], but we found that substantially extending this step confers only modest improvements in EV removal and may not impact whether FBS-derived EVs are present in substantial quantities in the conditioned medium at **step 4** (*see* Fig. 2 and **Note 1**).

5. Expression plasmid encoding EV membrane protein of interest fused to an affinity tag (tag-protein) compatible with affinity chromatography; we used the FLAG tag fused to Lamp2b. If the EV subset of interest is endosomally derived (exosomes),

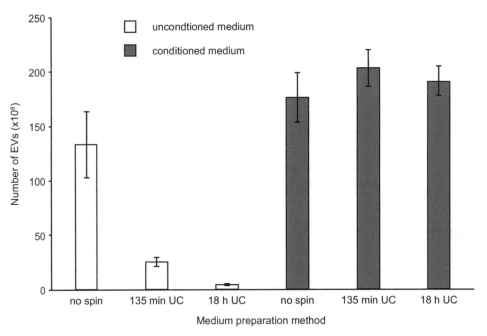

Fig. 2 EV yield as a function of EV depletion method. EV-depleted media were prepared by ultracentrifugation for various amounts of time (*see* Subheading 3.1, **step 3**), and residual EVs were quantified in these unconditioned media. The same media were also used to culture HEK293FT cells for 24 h, after which conditioned media were collected and EVs quantified. In each case, EV yields refer to the total number of EVs collected from a 15 cm plate of cells (or the corresponding volume of cell-free medium for unconditioned media samples). This experiment was conducted in technical triplicate and is representative of two independent experiments. Error bars indicate one standard deviation

it may be useful to protect the affinity tag from endosomal proteases by introducing an engineered glycosylation motif (*see* **Note 2**).

6. Transfection reagents compatible with the EV-producing cell line of interest. Transfections performed in this instance used a calcium phosphate transfection, which requires 2 M Calcium Chloride and 2× HEPES Buffered Saline Solution (HeBS) (280 mM NaCl, 1.5 mM Na_2HPO_4, 11.9 mg/mL HEPES, pH 7.1) stocks.

2.2 Affinity Chromatography

1. Anti-FLAG M2 affinity gel (Sigma).
2. 4 mL 1 × 5 cm glass chromatography column (BioRad).
3. Tris-Buffered Saline (TBS): 50 mM Tris–Cl, 150 mM NaCl, pH 7.5.
4. Regeneration buffer: 0.1 M glycine–HCl, pH 3.5.
5. Elution buffer: 3× FLAG peptide (Sigma) resuspended at 100 µg/mL in desired buffer; we validated elution with TBS or cell culture medium.
6. Storage buffer: 50% glycerol, 0.02% sodium azide in TBS.

2.3 EV Quantification

1. NanoSight LM10-HS (Malvern) with a laser wavelength of 405 nm and NanoSight NTA software v2.3, or similar instrument and software.
2. Calibration beads: 1:1000 100 nm calibration beads (Malvern) in TBS.
3. Ultrapure water: Milli-Q ultrapure water (EMD Millipore).

3   Methods

For all parts of the protocol involving cell culture, or when handling EVs to be used in downstream cell culture-based experiments, perform procedures in a BSL2 tissue culture biosafety cabinet and don appropriate personal protective equipment (e.g., lab coat, latex/nitrile gloves, safety glasses).

3.1 Display of Tag-Protein on the Surface of EVs

To isolate EVs expressing a protein of interest, it is necessary to transfect EV-producing cells with an affinity-tagged version of this protein which can be isolated by anti-tag affinity chromatography. In this instance of the method, we fused the FLAG tag to the extra-vesicular terminus of the late endosomal transmembrane protein, Lamp2b, which is incorporated into exosomes. If desired, this protocol could be adapted to use other affinity tags or other EV membrane proteins, although the biochemistry of such a system may need to be optimized to achieve efficient display of the tag on the vesicle surface. Whenever possible, in the discussion below, we highlight variables that can be tuned to impact the degree to which a peptide is displayed on the EV surface.

1. Create an expression plasmid in which the FLAG affinity tag (DYKDDDDK) is fused to the extra-vesicular terminus of an EV membrane protein. For details on the specific case of tagging Lamp2b, *see* **Note 2**.

2. Transfect the tag-protein expression plasmid generated in **step 1** into the chosen EV-producing cells. For recommendations on optimizing the transfection, *see* **Note 3**. 12–16 h after transfection of EV-producing cells, change medium to EV-depleted medium.

3. 24 h after medium change, harvest conditioned medium from EV-producing cells.

3.2 Isolation of EVs from Conditioned Medium of EV-Producing Cells

Steps **5–7** have been previously described [6]. For tips on EV storage conditions, *see* **Note 4**.

1. Centrifuge conditioned medium at 4 °C at $300 \times g$ for 10 min and retrieve the supernatant. This step clears the medium of cells.

2. Centrifuge the supernatant from **step 5** at $2000 \times g$ for 10 min and retrieve the supernatant. This step clears the medium of cell debris.

3. Optional, depending on EV population of interest: centrifuge the supernatant at $10,000 \times g$ for 30 min and retrieve the supernatant. This step clears the medium of apoptotic bodies and some microvesicles.

4. Prepare the anti-FLAG affinity column by loading 1.0 mL of anti-FLAG M2 affinity gel into a 4 mL 1×5 cm glass chromatography column and draining via gravity flow. If reusing a stored column, drain the storage buffer and continue to **step 9**. Do not let the resin run dry at any point.

5. Rinse the column with 5 mL Tris-buffered saline (TBS).

6. Equilibrate the column with three sequential 1 mL washes of regeneration buffer, followed by a wash with 5 mL TBS.

7. Load clarified EV-containing supernatant onto the column five times, collecting and reusing the flow-through each time (*see* **Note 5**). For larger sample volumes, consider attaching a compatible funnel to the column entrance.

8. Wash the column with 10 mL TBS.

9. For elution of EVs, add 2.5 mL of elution buffer and incubate 5 min at room temperature (~22 °C). We have validated both TBS (for EV analysis) and EV-depleted medium (for investi-

gating EV delivery to recipient cells) as viable elution buffer solvents.

10. Collect elution buffer in fractions of ~0.5 mL each: ~5 fractions (*see* **Note 6**).

11. Regenerate the column by washing with 3 mL regeneration buffer.

12. Store column in storage buffer at 4 °C.

3.3 Analyzing EVs after Elution

Profile EV size distributions and concentrations by NTA. Using a NanoSight LM10-HS (Malvern) with a laser wavelength of 405 nm and NanoSight NTA software v2.3, the following protocol enables EV quantification. EVs should be quantified before and after affinity chromatography if quantification of yield is desired. For examples of characterization of EVs isolated by this method, *see* **Note 6**.

1. Acquire videos at camera level 14 (this setting may vary by instrument). Use the attached thermometer if available. If not, set the temperature in the software as ambient temperature (22 °C) and use calibration beads to check that sizing is accurate. Adjust the temperature as needed to ensure calibration beads are sized properly.

2. Introduce samples manually. Between different samples, wash the platform 3× with ultrapure water. For tips on NanoSight use, *see* **Note 7**.

3. Analyze a minimum of three 30 s videos per sample. As needed, dilute EVs in TBS to keep concentrations between $1–10 \times 10^8$ particles/mL (the accurate range of the NanoSight). Analyze videos at a detection threshold of 7 (this setting may vary by instrument). The blur, minimum track length, and minimum expected particle size should be set automatically by the software.

4. Isolated EVs can then be characterized and used in any number of other experiments, including immunostaining analysis of EV contents (example in **Note 8**), EV-mediated delivery of biomolecules to cells (example in **Note 9**), flow cytometry, sequencing, etc.

4 Notes

1. It has been reported that fully removing bovine EVs from FBS-supplemented medium by ultracentrifugation may require spinning samples overnight [ ]. We found that increasing this step from 135 min to 18 h conferred only modest additional removal of FBS-derived EVs (Fig. 2, white bars). Moreover, when HEK293FT cells were cultured for 24 h in media in which FBS-derived EVs were removed to these varying degrees,

the resulting concentrations of EVs in the cell supernatant were indistinguishable (Fig. 2, grey bars). It is possible that the FBS-derived EVs were either consumed by the cells or were otherwise degraded over this period. In any event, we concluded that using the protocol described here, it is unlikely that any substantial number of EVs recovered from cell supernatant will be derived from FBS, regardless of which depletion protocol is used, and therefore a 135 min depletion may be sufficient.

2. In our characterization of this affinity purification protocol, we fused the FLAG tag to the N-terminus of Lamp2b. In this fusion protein, starting from the N-terminus, the first peptide is the Lamp2b signal peptide (MVCFRLFPVPGSGLVLVCLVL GAVRSYA). Next, insert the N-linked glycosylation motif GNSTM, which protects the FLAG tag from endosomal degradation during EV biogenesis []. Downstream of the GNSTM motif is a GSG spacer, followed by the FLAG peptide. Next, another spacer, GSGSGSGGSS is downstream of the FLAG peptide. Then, the Lamp2b protein is encoded. While not essential to this protocol, we added another GSG spacer and the peptide YPYDVPYA (HA affinity tag) at the C-terminus to enable further analysis of protein expression in EVs. In other instances, we fused the fluorescent protein dTomato in place of the HA tag to enable analysis of EV delivery to recipient cells. We have found that the format described here results in high expression of the FLAG fusion protein on EVs. We have observed that adjusting the length of the spacer peptides affects the amount of FLAG peptide (and HA peptide) that can be detected in EVs, indicating that spacer length may affect overall protein expression. When investigating the endosomally derived subset of EVs known as exosomes, FLAG peptide displayed on the surface of exosomes is exposed to the lumen of the endosome during exosome biogenesis []. In these cases, the GNSTM glycosylation motif can protect the FLAG peptide from endosomal degradation, and therefore we suggest investigating the inclusion of such a motif when studying exosomes.

3. High transfection efficiency is desired for this protocol, as tag-protein expression impacts the total number of EVs that can be isolated by affinity chromatography. We have observed that it is possible to increase the number of EVs isolated by transfecting more tag-protein expression plasmid into the EV-producing cells (Fig. 3). In HEK293FT cells, up to 30 μg of the 6295 bp expression vector can be transfected into cells plated at ~10^6 cells/mL in 15 cm dishes (20 mL medium). Higher levels of transfection may be possible but were not explored here. EVs produced from cells transfected with 30 μg of the tag-

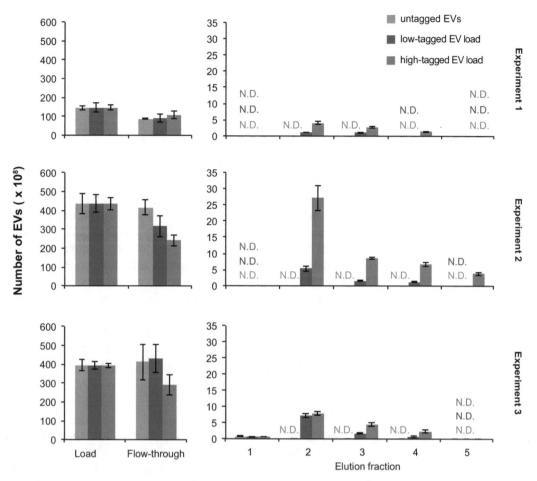

Fig. 3 Recovery of EVs from cell culture supernatant using affinity chromatography. Quantification of EV counts (by NanoSight analysis) observed in three independent trials of affinity chromatography-based EV isolation. Error bars indicate one standard deviation

protein expression vector were termed "high-tagged EVs" and appear in the red bars. Transfection of a lower amount of tag-protein expression vector (15 μg + 15 μg control plasmid with no expression cassette—"low-tagged EVs," blue bars) resulted in isolation of fewer EVs by affinity chromatography. As expected, EVs from non-transfected cells "untagged EVs" were detected in the load and flow-through, but not in the elution fractions (Fig. 3, gray bars). Notably, we observed a considerable degree of day-to-day variation in the number of EVs produced by the EV-producing cells (and therefore present in the load), as well as variation in the percent recovery of EVs by affinity chromatography. To provide the reader an accurate view of this variation, Fig. 3 presents the results of three independent EV generation and isolation experiments. It is not known whether these observations are limited to the HeBS-based calcium phosphate transfection method used in this study, or whether similar effects would be observed in the context of stable tag-protein expression or when using other transient transfection methods.

4. At any time, clarified conditioned medium can be stored at 4 °C for at least 48 h without loss of EVs. Purified EVs can be frozen at −80 °C without loss of EVs after one freeze-thaw cycle, although multiple freeze-thaw cycles are not recommended.

5. In our experience, loading the column by sequentially passing the conditioned medium over the column multiple times led to greater EV recovery, presumably by increasing contact time between the EVs and the affinity matrix. EV recovery following a single loading pass was minimal, and we typically observed diminishing returns between 3 and 5 passes over the column, such that five passes is a relatively robust general loading strategy. For EV preps in which tag presentation is less efficient, or in which different tag-antibody pairs are used, it may be useful to increase contact time between EVs and the affinity matrix (beads) by other methods. For example, beads may be preincubated with EVs prior to loading the column, EVs may be incubated with beads on the column, or a greater number of loading passes may be used.

6. As shown in Fig. 3, this affinity chromatography method recovers only a small fraction of the initial EV population that is present in conditioned medium. Low-tagged EVs were present in the load, flow-through, and elution fractions (Fig. 3, blue bars), and approximately 1.5–2.5% of low-tagged EVs loaded on the column were recovered in the elution fractions (Table 1). High-tagged EVs were also present in the load, flow-through, and elution fractions, but these EVs were consistently eluted to a greater extent than were low-tagged EVs (Fig. 3, red vs. blue bars). Approximately 5% of the loaded high-tagged EVs were recovered in the elution fractions (Table 1). Fractional elution is recommended, as the majority of column-bound EVs elute in a given fraction (Fig. 3). This property could vary depending on the purification tag used, or the amount of EVs present in the sample. Once this property is determined for a protocol, it is not necessary to collect fractions beyond the primary elution (in this case, fractions 3, 4, and 5 could be combined) unless increased recovery is desired. Additionally, elution buffer volume beyond what is required to elute the majority of column-bound EVs can be omitted to minimize consumption of costly elution reagents. The EV size distributions in the load and elution fractions were similar as measured by NTA, indicating that affinity chromatography did

Table 1
Quantification of EV recoveries for each affinity chromatography experiment shown in Fig. 3

	Percent recovery		
	Untagged EVs	Low-tagged EVs	High-tagged EVs
Experiment 1	N.D.	1.5	5.5
Experiment 2	N.D.	1.9	5.3
Experiment 3	0.19	2.6	3.9
Mean		*2.0*	*4.9*
Standard deviation		*0.57*	*0.86*

Percent recovery = (total count of EVs in the combined elution fractions)/(total count of EVs in the load fraction) × 100. The mean percent recovery for the low-tagged EV sample was not significantly different from the high-tagged EV sample, using a two-tailed Student's t-test ($p = 0.06$)

not significantly alter this property or enrich for a subset of any particular size (Fig. 4).

7. Before loading EV samples on the NanoSight platform, ensure that all screws are tight and the platform is evenly aligned. If this is not the case, sample will leak out of the platform, or the sample may drift during the video, preventing accurate sizing. Check by first loading a water sample and ensuring leakage does not occur. Load samples slowly and evenly with a 1 mL syringe to avoid bubble formation. It is important to minimize flow of sample in the platform as much as possible, as this can lead to inaccurate measurements. Leave the 1 mL syringe in the loading platform during video acquisition. If desired, sample can be removed from the NanoSight using the syringe. In case issues arise during acquisition, it is a good idea to retain the sample for subsequent analysis, if needed.

8. It may be of interest to investigate the degree to which affinity-isolated EVs are enriched in tag-protein. In our demonstration of this method, the tag-protein contains a second affinity tag (HA) on the EV luminal face, which was used for western blot analysis to avoid potential interference by FLAG peptide or anti-FLAG antibodies introduced during affinity chromatography. Equal numbers of low-tagged or high-tagged EVs purified by ultracentrifugation (the current "gold standard" in EV isolation) or affinity chromatography were analyzed (Fig. 5). Relative to the load, EVs in the elution fraction contained substantially more tag-protein. EVs in the elution fraction were also enriched in tag-protein relative to ultracentrifugation-isolated EVs. The enrichment was particularly evident for short

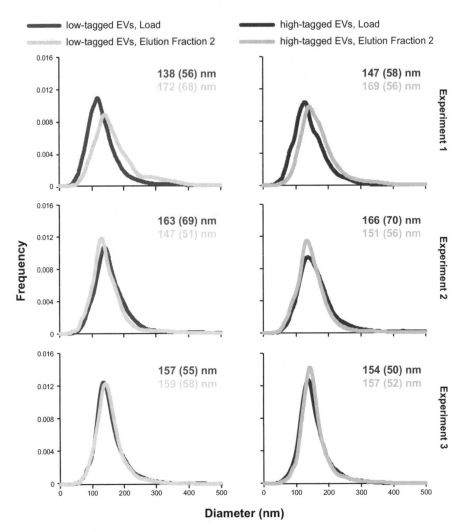

Fig. 4 Effect of affinity chromatographic recovery on EV size distributions. EV size distributions were quantified by NanoSight analysis in the load and elution fraction 2 (*see* Fig. 3) for low-tagged or high-tagged EVs. *Numbers inset* in each panel represent "Mean (StDev)" of each distribution

blot exposure times (Fig. 5, left). This enrichment was stronger for the low-tagged EVs than for the high-tagged EVs. To explain this observation, we hypothesize that when EV-producing cells express greater levels of the tag-protein, more of the EVs produced will express the tag-protein, and each EV produced may on average contain more tag-protein as well. This effect would explain why high-tagged EVs contained a similar amount of tag-protein, on average, independently of which purification method was used. While we expected EVs isolated by affinity chromatography to be enriched in tag-protein relative to the load, interestingly, a similar effect was observed for ultracentrifuge-isolated EVs. To explain this

L: Load
F: Flow-through
E: Eluted
U: Ultracentrifuged

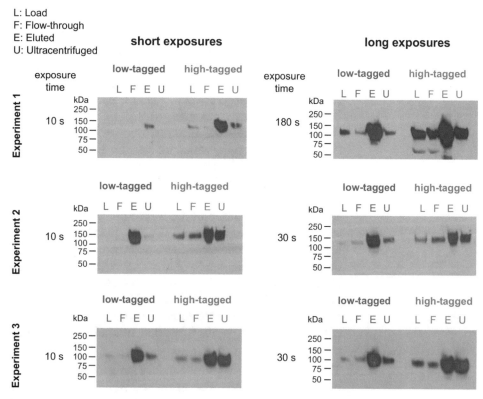

Fig. 5 Chromatographic enrichment of tagged EV subsets. Equal numbers of ultracentrifuge-purified EVs (U), or EVs from the load (L), flow-through (F), and elution fraction 2 (E) were loaded into each lane and analyzed by western blot against the C-terminal HA tag in the tag-protein. Both long and short exposures of each gel are included to highlight key features of these data. Short exposures demonstrated profound enrichment of tag-protein in the eluted EVs relative to the other samples, particularly in the case of low-tagged EVs. Long exposures indicated the presence of some tag-protein in all four samples

observation, we note that the ultracentrifugation protocol used here was optimized for isolation of exosomes, a subset of EVs that are endosomally derived and therefore likely to incorporate Lamp2b fusion proteins [10, 11]. Thus, the load fraction may contain a more heterogeneous mix of EVs (and therefore a lower average level of tag-protein expression) than would the ultracentrifuge-purified EVs. Overall, affinity purification of EVs substantially enhanced the amount of tag-protein per EV compared to either the load fraction or ultracentrifuge-purified EVs. For blotting tag-protein we used rabbit anti-HA antibody (Cell Signaling Technology C29F4) diluted 1:1000 and incubated overnight at 4 °C as a primary antibody. The secondary antibody used was horseradish peroxidase-conjugated goat-anti-rabbit immunoglobulin G secondary antibody (Thermo-Fisher Scientific).

9. We also observed that affinity-isolated EVs retain the ability to deliver protein to recipient cells. To track cargo delivery to recipient cells, EVs were generated from cells expressing a modified tag-protein in which the C-terminus (corresponding to the EV lumen) was fused to the dTomato fluorescent protein as a model cargo protein. These labeled EVs were isolated by either affinity chromatography or ultracentrifugation, counted, and delivered in equal numbers to prostate cancer (PC-3) recipient cells, which we previously observed to readily take up EVs [12]. Recipient PC-3 cells were plated 24–36 h before EV delivery at ~1.5 × 10^5 cells/mL in 48-well plates (0.5 mL medium). After 17 h of incubation with EVs, recipient cells were profiled by flow cytometry (Fig. 6). For both low-tagged and high-tagged EVs, isolation by affinity chromatography enhanced the extent to which cargo protein was delivered to recipient cells. Altogether, these data suggest that affinity chromatography may be harnessed to enhance the potency of EVs as cargo delivery vehicles by effectively increasing the average concentration of cargo molecules per vesicle, compared to EVs purified by conventional ultracentrifugation methods.

10. There are several avenues for further optimization of affinity purification of EVs. For example, while anti-FLAG affinity chromatography is convenient for research-scale EV isolation, other affinity chromatography systems could be useful for applications such as larger-scale EV production for therapeutic applications. We also observed that EVs in the flow-through fraction still contained some tag-protein (Fig. 5), indicating incomplete isolation of tag-protein containing EVs. One potential explanation for this phenomenon is column saturation, which may be a function of EV size. This study used commercially available conjugated agarose bead resin as a chromatography matrix, which is highly nanoporous. Since some EVs are larger in diameter than are the matrix nanopores, it is possible that the EVs did not have access to the internal binding capacity of the matrix, and thus there may exist fewer effective binding sites for tagged EVs than is the case for tagged recombinant proteins. Should this effect prove to be limiting, enhanced EV recovery could potentially be achieved by utilizing a macroporous and monolithic matrix, such as one prepared through cryogelation techniques [13]. Optimizing other chromatography conditions such as buffer and flow rate may also enhance EV yield to some extent. Beyond avoiding column saturation, scaling up EV yields may also benefit from pairing affinity separation with methods for generating higher starting concentrations of EVs, such as growing EV-producing cells in hollow-fiber bioreactors [14].

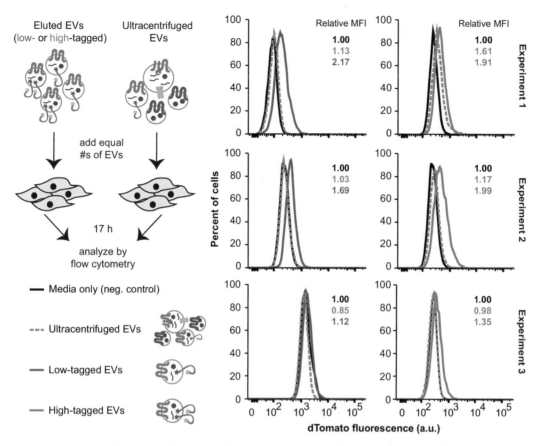

Fig. 6 Enhanced cargo protein delivery by chromatographically enriched EV subsets. *Left*: cartoon demonstrating experimental setup. Equal numbers of EVs or affinity chromatography eluted EVs containing glycosylated FLAG-Lamp2b-dTomato-HA fusion protein were administered to PC-3 recipient cells for 17 h. *Right*: fluorescence of recipient cells as measured by flow cytometry. *Numbers inset* in each panel represent the mean fluorescence intensity (MFI) of each sample normalized to the MFI of the negative control in the same experiment

Acknowledgements

Theint Aung and Dr. Arabela Grigorescu (Northwestern University) provided assistance with NanoSight analysis, which was performed at the Northwestern University Keck Biophysics Facility. Traditional sequencing services were performed at the Northwestern University Genomics Core Facility. Andrew Younger (Northwestern University) provided assistance with plasmid construction. This work was supported by a 3M Non-tenured Faculty Award, the Lynn Sage Breast Cancer Foundation and Northwestern Memorial Foundation, and the Northwestern University Prostate Cancer Specialized Program of Research Excellence (SPORE) through NIH award P50 CA090386 (to J.N.L.). This work was also supported by the National Science Foundation's Graduate Research Fellowship Program (NSF GRFP) award DGE-0824162 (to M.E.H.) and award DGE-1324585 (to D.M.S.). M.E.H. and J.N.L. are inventors on a US patent application covering inventions described in this manuscript.

References

1. Gyorgy B, Hung ME, Breakefield XO, Leonard JN (2015) Therapeutic applications of extracellular vesicles: clinical promise and open questions. Annu Rev Pharmacol Toxicol 55: 439–464. https://doi.org/10.1146/annurev-pharmtox-010814-124630

2. El-Andaloussi S, Mager I, Breakefield XO, Wood MJ (2013) Extracellular vesicles: biology and emerging therapeutic opportunities. Nat Rev Drug Discov 12(5):347–357. https://doi.org/10.1038/nrd3978

3. Gyorgy B, Szabo TG, Pasztoi M, Pal Z, Misjak P, Aradi B, Laszlo V, Pallinger E, Pap E, Kittel A, Nagy G, Falus A, Buzas EI (2011) Membrane vesicles, current state-of-the-art: emerging role of extracellular vesicles. Cell Mol Life Sci 68(16):2667–2688. https://doi.org/10.1007/s00018-011-0689-3

4. Smith ZJ, Lee C, Rojalin T, Carney RP, Hazari S, Knudson A, Lam K, Heikki S, Ibanez EL, Viitala T, Laaksonen T, Yliperttula M, Wachsmann-Hogiu S (2015) Single exosome study reveals subpopulations distributed among cell lines with variability related to membrane content. J Extracell Vesicles 4:28533

5. Willms E, Johansson HJ, Mager I, Lee Y, Blomberg KE, Sadik M, Alaarg A, Smith CI, Lehtio J, El Andaloussi S, Wood MJ, Vader P (2016) Cells release subpopulations of exosomes with distinct molecular and biological properties. Sci Rep 6:22519. https://doi.org/10.1038/srep22519

6. Thery C, Amigorena S, Raposo G, Clayton A (2006) Isolation and characterization of exosomes from cell culture supernatants and biological fluids. Curr Protoc Cell Biol/editorial board, Juan S. Bonifacino [et al.] Chapter 3:Unit 3.22. https://doi.org/10.1002/0471143030.cb0322s30

7. Mathivanan S, Lim JW, Tauro BJ, Ji H, Moritz RL, Simpson RJ (2010) Proteomics analysis of A33 immunoaffinity-purified exosomes released from the human colon tumor cell line LIM1215 reveals a tissue-specific protein signature. Mol Cell Proteomics 9(2):197–208. https://doi.org/10.1074/mcp.M900152-MCP200

8. Hung ME, Leonard JN (2015) Stabilization of exosome-targeting peptides via engineered glycosylation. J Biol Chem 290(13):8166–8172. https://doi.org/10.1074/jbc.M114.621383

9. Witwer KW, Buzas EI, Bemis LT, Bora A, Lasser C, Lotvall J, Nolte-'t Hoen EN, Piper MG, Sivaraman S, Skog J, Thery C, Wauben MH, Hochberg F (2013) Standardization of sample collection, isolation and analysis methods in extracellular vesicle research. J Extracell Vesicles 2. https://doi.org/10.3402/jev.v2i0.20360

10. Alvarez-Erviti L, Seow Y, Yin H, Betts C, Lakhal S, Wood MJ (2011) Delivery of siRNA to the mouse brain by systemic injection of targeted exosomes. Nat Biotechnol 29(4):341–345. https://doi.org/10.1038/nbt.1807

11. Caby MP, Lankar D, Vincendeau-Scherrer C, Raposo G, Bonnerot C (2005) Exosomal-like vesicles are present in human blood plasma. Int Immunol 17(7):879–887. https://doi.org/10.1093/intimm/dxh267

12. Hung ME, Leonard JN (2016) A platform for actively loading cargo RNA to elucidate limiting steps in EV-mediated delivery. J Extracell Vesicles 5:31027

13. Reichelt S (2015) Introduction to macroporous cryogels. Methods Mol Biol 1286:173–181. https://doi.org/10.1007/978-1-4939-2447-9_14

14. Whitford W, Ludlow J, Cadwell J (2015) Continuous production of exosomes: utilizing the technical advantages of hollow-fiber bioreactor technology. Genet Eng Biotechnol News 35(16):34. https://doi.org/10.1089/gen.35.16.15

Chapter 10

Detection and Analysis of Non-vesicular Extracellular RNA

Juan Pablo Tosar and Alfonso Cayota

Abstract

Although extracellular vesicles (EVs) are by far the most studied carriers of extracellular small RNAs involved in cell-to-cell communication, most extracellular small RNAs are actually present as soluble vesicle-free supramolecular complexes. Several proteins have been described as the counterparts of these RNase-protected complexes. Here we describe a method for the purification and analysis of non-vesicular extracellular RNA derived from the conditioned media of mammalian cell culture. Focus on this fraction will increase our understanding on extracellular RNA biology, while serving as a source for biomarker discovery complementary to EVs.

Key words Exosomes, Ribonucleoprotein fraction, miRNA, tRNA fragments, Sequencing

1 Introduction

There is growing interest in profiling extracellular RNA (exRNA), especially after the first reports describing transfer of functional regulatory RNAs between nonadjacent cells [1–3]. On the other hand, the fact that cells secrete a fraction of their transcriptome to the extracellular space has attracted great attention because it offers a way of performing disease-associated biomarker analysis in minimally invasive liquid biopsies [4].

Extracellular vesicles (EVs) protect RNAs against the action of extracellular RNases, and bare a number of surface-exposed adhesion molecules which mediate EV uptake by specific cell types [5]. For these reasons, EVs were initially thought to be the main source of exRNA and the physiological vectors for regulatory RNA exchange between cells. However, stoichiometric analysis has shown that the miRNA content of exosomes is not as high as previously thought, with no more than a copy of any single miRNA per exosome, in average [6]. On the other hand, the vast majority of RNase-protected circulating miRNAs in serum was reported to be present in ribonucleoprotein complexes [7]. The extracellular miRNA-binding proteins include

Tushar Patel (ed.), *Extracellular RNA: Methods and Protocols*, Methods in Molecular Biology, vol. 1740,
https://doi.org/10.1007/978-1-4939-7652-2_10, © Springer Science+Business Media, LLC 2018

nucleophosmin 1 [8] and the catalytic core of the miRNA-induced silencing complex, Argonaute 2 [7, 9].

We have performed comparative analysis of the extracellular small RNA content present in serum-free cultures of breast cell lines, including EV and non-EV (i.e., ribonucleoprotein) fractions [10]. Our results showed profound enrichment of tRNA halves, a recently discovered family of regulatory RNAs with varied functions [11–13], in the ribonucleoprotein fraction. Thus, a comprehensive analysis of the extracellular RNA content needs to consider the pool of RNAs not associated with EVs, which seems to be the major reservoir of miRNAs and other small RNA species, at least under certain experimental conditions.

Herein, we detail a protocol for extracellular small RNA profiling of non-vesicular RNA, extracted from conditioned cell culture media. Most researchers in the EV-associated RNA field use vesicle-depleted fetal bovine serum (10%) in the complete medium formulation. This is typically achieved by performing long (> 12 h) ultracentrifugation (>100,000 × g at 4 °C) of fetal bovine serum in order to pellet serum-associated EVs. However, this protocol will not eliminate serum-associated ribonucleoprotein complexes, which would interfere in the analysis. Readers should be aware that miRNAs and noncoding RNAs tend to be highly conserved in mammals, making most bovine small RNAs indistinguishable from their human counterparts (in case the analysis is performed in human cell lines). Thus, we highly recommend growing the cell lines under defined formulations to avoid misinterpretations of results by contaminating vesicle-free RNAs from serum (*see* **Note 1**).

This protocol is intended for profiling small RNAs by next generation sequencing, though sequencing-related protocols are beyond the scope of this chapter. Although the protocol includes a chromatographic step (in order to focus in more specific populations), RNA extraction can be performed after ultracentrifugation to achieve a more representative scenario of the extracellular small RNAome. However, most of the reads will probably correspond to ncRNA fragments and not miRNAs [10].

2 Materials

Prepare all solutions using sterile nuclease-free water. Reagents should be analytical grade and suitable for molecular biology, and RNase-free certified. Keep aseptic techniques and appropriate laboratory practices for cell culture, and take adequate precautions to minimize RNase contamination during the whole process. Especially, use clean gloves whenever handling samples and disposable single-use materials whenever possible. Clean the lab bench and the micropipettes with RNase decontaminating solutions before use, and use micropipette tips with filters to avoid contamination by aerosol formation. Keep conditioned media and purified RNA in ice during handling.

2.1 Cell Culture

1. Human breast cancer cell line MCF-7 obtained from a certified repository (e.g., ATCC). Other cell lines can be used, but the culture protocol should be adapted to match the specific cell requirements.

2. Complete growth medium: Eagle's Minimum Essential Medium (EMEM) containing 0.01 mg/mL recombinant human insulin and 10% fetal bovine serum.

3. Sterile Dulbecco's Phosphate Buffered Saline (DPBS): 1.47 mM KH_2PO_4, 8.06 mM $Na_2HPO_4 \cdot 7H_2O$, 2.67 mM KCl, 137.93 mM NaCl.

4. Sterile 0.05% Trypsin-EDTA solution.

5. Defined Serum-free medium: EMEM containing 3.8 μg/mL recombinant human insulin, 0.8 ng/mL Epidermal Growth Factor (EGF), 5 μg/mL human Transferrin, 475 pg/ml Prostaglandin F2alpha (PGF2α), and 20 μg/mL Fibronectin.

6. Trypan blue solution, 0.4%.

7. Murine RNase inhibitor.

2.2 Conditioned Media Fractionation

1. Refrigerated ultracentrifuge with swinging-bucket rotor capable of achieving at least $100,000 \times g$.

2. Ultracentrifugation tubes (14 mL). If possible, use disposable tubes not previously used before.

3. Ultrafiltration tubes (20 mL) with a molecular weight cutoff (MWCO) ≤ 10 kDa.

2.3 RNA Purification

1. Nuclease-free tubes and tips (with filter).

2. RNase decontaminating solution for surfaces.

3. Trizol® LS (liquid sample) reagent.

4. Chloroform, anhydrous (≥99%).

5. Isopropyl alcohol (2-propanol), suitable for molecular biology (>99.5%).

6. Nuclease-free glycogen, suitable for nucleic acid precipitations.

7. 80% ethanol solution (prepared with nuclease-free water).

8. Qubit RNA high-sensitivity (HS) Kit (Thermo).

9. Bioanalyzer small RNA kit (Agilent). A high-sensitivity DNA kit will be later used for quality-control of next generation sequencing libraries.

10. Kits for small RNA next generation sequencing (library preparation + sequencing reactions). Follow manufacturer's instructions (sequencing library preparation goes beyond the scope of this protocol).

2.4 Chromatographic Fractionation of 100,000 × g Supernatants

1. Superdex 75 10/300 column and Äkta FPLC system (GE).
2. Sterile 1 mL syringe and needle.
3. Clean 96-well fractionation plates.
4. 0.22 μm-filtered and degassed solutions (500 mL): DEPC-treated water, nuclease-free or DEPC-treated DPBS, and ethanol 20%.

3 Methods

3.1 Collection of Cell Conditioned Media

The specific protocols for this section may vary according to the requirements of the cell lines under study. For explanatory reasons, we will use the adherent breast cancer cell line MCF-7 (ATCC HTB-22), which we routinely use in our lab.

All procedures should be performed in a laminar-flow cell culture cabin, in laboratories with adequate biosafety levels for the cell line under study (BSL1 for MCF-7). Readers are supposed to have basic experience with mammalian cell culture.

1. Identify a frozen ampule stored in liquid nitrogen, or purchase an ampule directly from a certified supplier. Frozen ampules should be used at low passage (<10) for greater reproducibility (*see* **Notes 2** and **3**).
2. Thaw the ampule (containing approx. 1×10^6 cells) and immediately dilute in a sterile plastic tube containing at least 5 mL of pre-warmed (37 °C) complete growth medium (*see* **Note 4**).
3. Centrifuge the cells at $300 \times g$ for 5 min at room temperature. Go back to the biosafety cabinet and gently remove the supernatant. Add 6 mL of pre-warmed complete growth medium and gently aspirate the cell suspension with a sterile pipette.
4. Transfer the cell suspension to a 75 cm² cell culture flask, containing 4 mL of pre-warmed complete growth medium. Label the flask and incubate overnight at 37 °C in a CO_2 incubator (air, 95%; CO_2, 5%).
5. Remove the medium (containing nonattached cells) and supplement with 10 mL of pre-warmed complete growth medium. Incubate the cells for 48 h (*see* **Note 5**).
6. Repeat the previous step until a confluence of approx. 80%. Do not let cells become 100% confluent (*see* **Note 6**).

7. Remove culture medium, and immediately wash the cells with 5–10 mL of pre-warmed sterile DPBS. Remove the washing solution, and add 3 mL of a pre-warmed sterile Trypsin-EDTA solution. Place the cells in the CO_2 incubator for 5 min, and observe under an inverted microscope until the cell layer is dispersed. If a significant number of cells are still attached to the plastic, incubate for additional 5–10 min. Remove the Trypsin-EDTA solution containing the detached cells, and dilute in a plastic tube containing 6 mL of pre-warmed complete growth medium. Take a small aliquot (<0.5 mL) to perform cell count in a Neubauer chamber (ideally following vital colorant staining). Centrifuge the tube containing the cells at $300 \times g$ for 5 min at room temperature.

8. Remove the supernatant, and gently resuspend the cells in an adequate volume of pre-warmed complete growth medium. Transfer 1×10^6 cells to two 75 cm² culture flasks. Complete the volume (10 mL) with pre-warmed complete growth medium, and incubate overnight at 37 °C.

9. Gently remove the medium, and wash the cells twice with 5 mL of pre-warmed sterile DPBS. Remove the washing solution, and add 10 mL of defined serum-free medium (*see* **Notes 7 and 8**). Incubate at 37 °C for 48 h.

10. Remove and discard the cell conditioned medium. Wash with pre-warmed DPBS, remove the washing solution, and add 10 mL of pre-warmed defined serum-free medium (*see* **Note 9**). Incubate for further 48 h.

11. Observe the cells under an inverted microscope. The percentage of detached cells should be low and similar to the one obtained after 48 h in serum-containing medium (it is advisable to run this control in parallel). Adhered cells should look viable, although we routinely observe slight changes in morphology. Cell confluence should be 70–80% (*see* **Note 10**).

12. Collect the cell conditioned medium from both flasks (20 mL) and add 80 U of murine RNase inhibitor. Centrifuge for 5 min at $800 \times g$ to remove remnant cells. Store the tube containing the supernatant at −20 °C for up to a month (*see* **Note 11**).

13. While centrifuging the conditioned media, detach cells with Trypsin-EDTA and perform cell count with vital staining (i.e., Trypan Blue). The percentage of viable cells should be high (>95%) and the cell's duplication time should be comparable to the one obtained with complete growth medium (*see* **Note 12**).

3.2 Conditioned Media Fractionation

1. Thaw the tube containing the cell-free conditioned medium at room temperature, with recurrent and very gentle inversion of the tube for even defrost. As soon as the last macroscopic evidence of ice is vanished, place in a precooled (4 °C) centrifuge, and

centrifuge at $2000 \times g$ for 20 min in a swinging-bucket rotor. Immediately transfer the supernatant to a new tube and keep on ice (*see* **Note 13**).

2. Divide the supernatant (20 mL) in two ultracentrifuge tubes. Adjust the volume with sterile DPBS to achieve the tube's optimal volume. Equilibrate both tubes in an analytical balance. Fill with water and equilibrate as many tubes as needed to complete the number of ultracentrifugation tubes admitted by the rotor. Mass differences between equilibrated tubes should be below 2 mg. Use calibrated micropipettes for equilibration. Always split the conditioned media to equilibrate tubes. Do not equilibrate conditioned media with water (*see* **Note 14**).

3. Place the rotor in the centrifuge and start the vacuum. Centrifuge at least at $100,000 \times g$ for 2.5 h at 4 °C (*see* **Note 15**).

4. Transfer the supernatant to a new tube. Keep the pellet if analysis of extracellular vesicles is also intended (*see* **Note 16**).

3.3 Concentration of the 100,000 × g Supernatant

1. Take a new ultrafiltration tube with a volume of 20 mL and a molecular weight cutoff (MWCO) of 10 kDa or lower (and a second one for equilibration). Add 10 mL of filtered ultrapure water, pipette up and down for several times with a p1000 micropipette twice, and centrifuge in a swinging-bucket rotor at the maximum allowed speed ($5000 \times g$ for Vivaspin 20 concentrators) for 10 min at 4 °C (*see* **Note 17**). Make sure all water has flowed from the concentration chamber to the lower chamber. Otherwise, increase centrifugation time.

2. Discard the flow-through and transfer the conditioned media's $100,000 \times g$ supernatant to the upper chamber of the ultrafiltration tube. Centrifugate at 4 °C until the remaining volume in the upper chamber is approximately 0.25 mL (0.5 mL if proceeding to size-exclusion chromatography). Stop centrifugation every 10 min and homogenate the concentrate by gently pipetting back and forth with a clean tip.

3. Proceed directly to RNA extraction (Subheading 3.4) or continue through the next steps before proceeding to the chromatographic separation of soluble RNA complexes (Subheading 3.5).

4. Gently dilute the concentrate with 10 mL of filtered DPBS, and concentrate again. This will change the sample matrix from EMEM (containing phenol red and other low molecular weight compounds) to DPBS. Macromolecules (including small RNAs) will remain in the concentrate.

5. Repeat the previous step once. Concentrate until the volume is 0.5 mL.

3.4 RNA Purification

1. Transfer the concentrate from **step 2** in Subheading 3.3 (0.25 mL) to a 1.5 mL clean Eppendorf tube. Add 0.75 mL of Trizol LS (if the starting volume is different from 0.25 mL,

keep the 3:1 volumetric ratio). Mix and let the tube stand at room temperature for 10 min to ensure dissociation of nucleoprotein complexes. Samples can be safely stored at –20 °C for later use (or at 4 °C overnight). Make sure to homogenate by successive inversions of the tube after thawing (*see* **Note 18**).

2. Add 0.2 mL of chloroform, and vigorously mix by successive inversions of the tube. The sample should turn its color from red to pink, and small droplets of water should immediately start to form. Let tubes stand at room temperature for 10 min. By that time, phase separation should be obvious. The upper colorless aqueous phase contains the RNA, while the lower red-colored organic phase contains denatured proteins. A white interphase is often observed in these samples (*see* **Note 19**).

3. Centrifuge at 12,000 × g and 4 °C for 15 min in a refrigerated table-top centrifuge. This will ensure complete phase separation.

4. Transfer 80–90% of the volume of the aqueous phase to a new tube. Make sure the interphase was not disturbed during the process (*see* **Notes 20** and **21**).

5. Add 5 μg of RNase-free glycogen, which will act as a carrier and will aid in RNA precipitation. Add at least 0.5 mL of RNase-free isopropyl alcohol to precipitate RNAs. Let the tubes stand at room temperature for 10 min. Then, centrifuge at 12,000 × g for 15 min at 4 °C.

6. Discard the supernatant. Add 1 mL of 80% ethanol to wash the pellet, which is probably not visible. Tilt the tube several times, until a small white pellet detaches from the bottom and slowly decants (*see* **Note 22**).

7. Centrifuge at 7500 × g for 5 min at 4 °C. Discard the supernatant. Place the tubes upside down over a clean sheet of absorbent paper for 10 min, in order to eliminate remaining ethanol droplets. Then, air-dry the pellets for further 10 min. Make sure ethanol droplets are no longer visible in the periphery of the pellet, but do not allow it to dry completely as this could make resuspension difficult.

8. Resuspend the pellet in 8 μL of RNase-free water. Use 1 μL for RNA quantification, and the remaining 7 μL for next generation sequencing library preparation (*see* **Note 23**).

3.5 Fractionation of the 100,000 × g Supernatants by Size-Exclusion Chromatography

1. Connect a Superdex 75 10/300 size-exclusion chromatography column to a fast protein liquid chromatography (FPLC) system. Fill the column with 30 mL of 0.22 μm-filtered and degassed water, and then equilibrate with an equal volume of 0.22 μm-filtered and degassed DPBS. Remember to set the pressure alarm at the maximum allowed pressure of the column (1.5 MPa). Install a 0.5 mL sample loop, and with the

help of a syringe fill the loop with DPBS. Keep the syringe at the injection point to avoid the entrance of air to the system.

2. Centrifuge the concentrate of **step 5** in Subheading 3.3 at 10,000 × g for 10 min at 4 °C. Transfer the supernatant to a new tube and aspire it with a sterile disposable 1 mL syringe. Remove the needle, face the syringe looking upwards, and move the plunger back and forth to eliminate any air bubbles between the plunger and the syringe's end.

3. Start a new run from the FPLC controller software. Set the pressure limit and a flow rate of 0.5 mL/min. Turn on the 280 and 260 nm detectors and perform an "auto zero" to set the baseline. Remove the buffer-containing syringe from the loop while gently pushing the plunger forward in order to keep the connector between the syringe and the loop filled with liquid. Immediately inject the sample, and change the injection valve from "load" to "inject." This will redirect the content of the loop to the chromatographic column.

4. Place a clean 96-well collection plate in the fractionator, and start collecting fractions of 0.2 mL. Stop the run after 30 mL post injection. Cover the collection and save it at 4 °C (*see* **Note 24**).

5. Pass 30 mL of filtered water to the column, and an equal volume of filtered 20% ethanol. Remove the column as indicated by the manufacturer in order to avoid entrance of air by any of the extremes.

6. Analyze the chromatogram. No increase in UV absorbance should be appreciable before the column exclusion volume (approximately 7.8 mL after injection). In general, the absorbance at 280 nm should be slightly higher than the absorbance at 260 nm, since the molar extinction coefficient of pure proteins has a maximum at 280 nm. Plot the 260/280 against the elution volume. Peaks in this plot might correspond to the elution of RNA (which has a maximum absorbance at 260 nm). We routinely observe ratios of 260/280 higher to 1 at 10.5 mL and 12.0 mL, and we have shown that these peaks correspond to tRNA halves [10] (Fig. 1).

7. If knowing what to look for, analyze each fraction of the eluate by specific assays. For example, perform Western Blot analysis to identify the fractions containing Argonaute2 (in order to sequence the Ago2-bound miRNAs) or stem-loop RT-qPCR to identify a specific miRNA. Go to the identified fractions and proceed to RNA purification (Subheading 3.4).

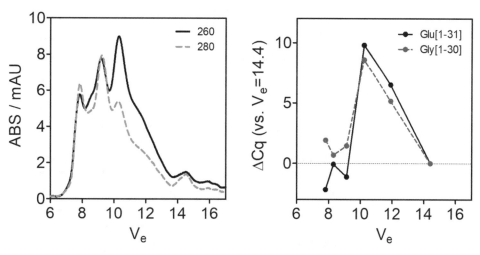

Fig. 1 The 100,000 × *g* supernatant from MCF-7 conditioned media was injected in a Superdex 75 10/300 column (size-exclusion chromatography) and fractions (200 μL) were eluted in DPBS using an ÄKTA purifier FPLC system (Amersham, GE Healthcare). *Left*: The chromatograms correspond to the absorbance at 280 nm (*gray dashed line*) and 260 nm (*black line*). V_e: elution volume. *Right*: Eluted fractions were assayed for the presence of 5′ halves from $tRNA_{Glu}^{CUC}$ (*black*) and $tRNA_{Gly}^{GCC}$ (*gray*) by stem-loop RT-qPCR. Cq values were compared to elution volume = 14.4 mL (where elution of tRNA-derived fragments is no longer expected)

---

4   Notes

1. An alternative is to grow the cells with EV-depleted fetal bovine serum, and sequence in parallel the nonconditioned complete growth medium.

2. In case of purchasing an ampule directly from a supplier such as the American Type Culture Collection (ATCC), store it immediately in liquid nitrogen indefinitely, or in a −70 °C refrigerator for up to 1 week. Before following this protocol, expand the cell line under optimal conditions (stated by the supplier) and obtain several ampules for liquid nitrogen storage. Supplier's instructions should be carefully followed for freezing (DMSO concentration, etc.).

3. The number of passages should be counted from the first time the ampules were thawed upon receipt (not the number of passages after the ampule was thawed from the researcher's backup stored in liquid nitrogen). Avoid using cell lines obtained from a collaborator unless strict control of the number of passages and freeze-thaw cycles can be supplied. If the ampule's history cannot be confidently tracked back to the original purchase, we recommend to avoid its use. Frozen ampules with an unknown record might contain contaminating cells, highly mutated genomes which significantly differ from the cell line's

original (especially for cancer cell lines passed several times), and microbial (especially *Mycoplasma*) contamination.

4. We strongly advise the use of serum-free media. However, we have found that MCF-7 cells won't adhere to the plastic with the supplied defined medium formulation. For this reason, we grow the cells with serum-containing media (no EV-depletion protocol) until achieving a desired number. Cells are then detached, subcultured, washed, and changed to serum-free conditions. We do not add antibiotics or antimycotics to culture media. Microbial contamination should be avoided by adequate handling and usage of sterile, disposable consumables. If microbial contamination is detected, discard all cells and working solutions and thaw a new ampule from the backup storage.

5. ATCC recommends transferring floating cells at the first two subcultures. We follow their protocol for the first two subcultures after purchasing the cells, but not after thawing backup ampules stored in liquid nitrogen.

6. MCF-7 cells grow in monolayer, but retain the ability to form domes.

7. All additives should be prepared sterile. We recommend diluting stock reactants with appropriate sterile solvents in a laminar flow cabinet. Be aware that 0.22 µM filtration of non-sterile solutions does not remove *Mycoplasma*.

8. We have also obtained good results for MCF-7 culture with a commercial serum-free medium, optimized for breast-derived cell lines: Mammary Epithelial Growth Medium (MEGM; Lonza). We do not add the Bovine Pituitary Extract contained in the kit, in order to keep a defined and controlled formulation. An advantage of this formulation is the lack of Transferrin, which can interfere in certain downstream assays (e.g., identification of RNAs which co-elute with Transferrin in size-exclusion chromatography).

9. We think it is appropriate to adapt cells to serum-free culture conditions before collection of cell conditioned media. This is the reason why we suggest discarding the conditioned media arising from the first 48 h. Besides, this conditioned media comes from a lower number of cells in comparison with the one collected in Subheading 3.1, **step 12**.

10. Lower confluences imply fewer cells, meaning less extracellular RNA in the conditioned media. If the number of cells is low, repeat the protocol by seeding a higher number of cells. Avoid conditioning media for longer than 48 h, because nutrient supplies start to decline, affecting cell viability.

11. We have found profound changes in the RNA profile of the conditioned media with or without addition of RNase inhibitor at this step. There are a number of brands commercializing recombinant human RNase inhibitor, but this protein is very sensible to oxidation and usually requires addition of 1 mM DTT. Murine RNase inhibitor is reportedly less sensible to oxidation and we do not add reducing agents at this step.

12. Nucleic acid fragmentation is often observed under stress (apoptosis being the extreme case) so stress-induced changes in the intracellular (small) RNA profile are expected, with predictable alterations of the extracellular RNAome. We tried to optimize culture conditions to keep the number of apoptotic cells to the minimum, but we cannot affirm that adaptation to serum-free culture does not impose any source of stress to the cells.

13. This will eliminate cell debris and eventual precipitates formed during the freeze-thaw process.

14. The ultracentrifuge and rotor should be cooled at 4 °C before use. The rotor should be preferentially placed in a refrigerator the night before or several hours before use. In our lab, we use a Beckman Coulter Optima XPN-90 ultracentrifuge and a SW40 Ti swinging-bucket rotor (k-factor = 137) with 14 mL thin wall Ultraclear disposable tubes. We do not reuse the tubes to avoid contamination of the samples.

15. Repeat this step to remove remaining extracellular vesicles from the supernatant.

16. If extracellular vesicles must be analyzed in parallel, resuspend the pellet in a low volume of DPBS by vigorous pipetting back and forth with a micropipette (and using the tip to scratch the bottom of the tube) or by gentle vortexing. Then complete the volume of the tube with DPBS, and centrifuge again at 100,000 × g. Resuspend the washed pellet in a desired volume of DPBS or appropriate buffer, and proceed to downstream applications. Extracellular vesicles purified with this protocol will be a heterogeneous mix of exosomes and microvesicles, so avoid the term "exosomes" when describing this preparation.

17. Fixed-angle rotors can be used, but the tubes must be filled with lower volumes (14 mL instead of 20 mL), so refilling of the ultrafiltration tubes during concentration should be carried out. In principle, any refrigerated centrifuge compatible with 50 mL Falcon tubes can be used.

18. Trizol LS is a concentrated variant of the popular Trizol reagent, suitable for liquid samples instead of pellets. Make sure the final dilution of the reagent is the appropriate, by keeping the 3:1 volumetric ratio. We have found that contaminated Trizol is a source of contaminating reads in next generation sequencing,

so we recommend taking a small working aliquot instead of introducing micropipette tips inside the bottle.

19. We have found that after addition of Trizol LS to the concentrated $100,000 \times g$ supernatants, the samples usually turn brown or yellowish instead of red. This is because the presence of phenol red in the samples (it can be easily removed by following **steps 4** and **5** in Subheading 3.3 before RNA extraction). Phenol Red is a pH indicator which turns from red to yellow after acidification of the medium.

20. After addition of Trizol LS, the samples are RNase-safe, because Trizol contains chaotropic agents which denature RNases together with any other proteins in the sample. However, from this step onwards, RNase contamination can degrade the sample in seconds.

21. Incline the tube at an angle of 45° for easier aspiration of the aqueous phase. Do not try to take as much of the aqueous phase as possible, as this will benefit from a small increase in the RNA yield at the expense of a higher phenol contamination.

22. The manufacturer recommends washing the pellet with 75% ethanol. We have slightly increased this percentage because small RNases are significantly more soluble than large RNAs, and do not precipitate in diluted ethanol. However, we do not have empirical evidence to state the relevance of this variation.

23. RNA quantification is not straightforward. UV absorbance spectrum (obtained with a Nanodrop spectrophotometer) will probably show the convolution of two peaks at 260 and 270 nm. An absorbance maximum of 270 nm is indicative of the presence of phenol (contained in the Trizol formulation), which is partitioned between the aqueous and the organic phase. Thus, RNA concentration based on 260 nm absorbance might be highly overestimated. We recommend to use a Qubit fluorometric assay (Thermo Fisher) to quantitate the RNA, if available. However, RNA concentration estimated from 1 μL might be below the limit of detection of the assay. The best alternative is to perform an Agilent Bioanalyzer analysis of the RNA with a small RNA chip, which will give both an estimation of concentration and size-distribution. The minimum RNA quantities for small RNA next generation sequencing library preparation (as stated by the manufacturer of the kits under use) might not be achieved, without this being necessarily a problem. Such quantities are calculated for intracellular transcriptomes, where most of the RNA corresponds to large ribosomal RNAs. Extracellular samples should be thought as intrinsically enriched in small RNAs. This is also the reason why we perform RNA extraction directly with Trizol LS, without specific protocols for small RNA enrichment. Size-selection

is later performed by polyacrylamide gel electrophoresis of PCR-amplified DNA libraries obtained from non-fractionated total RNA.

24. Do not wait until the run is complete to remove the collection plate and save it in the fridge, if the elution volume of the desired RNA fraction is known beforehand from previous experiments. FPLC systems installed in cold rooms are the ideal situation.

Acknowledgments

This work was supported by Agencia Nacional de Investigación e Inovación (ANII, Uruguay), grant number FCE 2011 I 6159.

References

1. Valadi H, Ekstrom K, Bossios A, Sjostrand M, Lee JJ et al (2007) Exosome-mediated transfer of mRNAs and microRNAs is a novel mechanism of genetic exchange between cells. Nat Cell Biol 9:654–659

2. Pegtel DM, Cosmopoulos K, Thorley-Lawson DA, van Eijndhoven MA, Hopmans ES et al (2010) Functional delivery of viral miRNAs via exosomes. Proc Natl Acad Sci U S A 107:6328–6333

3. Skog J, Wurdinger T, van Rijn S, Meijer DH, Gainche L et al (2008) Glioblastoma microvesicles transport RNA and proteins that promote tumour growth and provide diagnostic biomarkers. Nat Cell Biol 10:1470–1476

4. Cortez MA, Bueso-Ramos C, Ferdin J, Lopez-Berestein G, Sood AK et al (2011) MicroRNAs in body fluids—the mix of hormones and biomarkers. Nat Rev Clin Oncol 8:467–477

5. Hoshino A, Costa-Silva B, Shen TL, Rodrigues G, Hashimoto A et al (2015) Tumour exosome integrins determine organotropic metastasis. Nature 527:329–335

6. Chevillet JR, Kang Q, Ruf IK, Briggs HA, Vojtech LN et al (2014) Quantitative and stoichiometric analysis of the microRNA content of exosomes. Proc Natl Acad Sci U S A 111:14888–14893

7. Arroyo JD, Chevillet JR, Kroh EM, Ruf IK, Pritchard CC et al (2011) Argonaute2 complexes carry a population of circulating microRNAs independent of vesicles in human plasma. Proc Natl Acad Sci U S A 108:5003–5008

8. Wang K, Zhang S, Weber J, Baxter D, Galas DJ (2010) Export of microRNAs and microRNA-protective protein by mammalian cells. Nucleic Acids Res 38:7248–7259

9. Turchinovich A, Weiz L, Langheinz A, Burwinkel B (2011) Characterization of extracellular circulating microRNA. Nucleic Acids Res 39:7223–7233

10. Tosar JP, Gámbaro F, Sanguinetti J, Bonilla B, Witwer KW et al (2015) Assessment of small RNA sorting into different extracellular fractions revealed by high-throughput sequencing of breast cell lines. Nucleic Acids Res 43(11):5601–5616

11. Honda S, Loher P, Shigematsu M, Palazzo JP, Suzuki R et al (2015) Sex hormone-dependent tRNA halves enhance cell proliferation in breast and prostate cancers. Proc Natl Acad Sci U S A 112:E3816–E3825

12. Ivanov P, Emara MM, Villen J, Gygi SP, Anderson P (2011) Angiogenin-induced tRNA fragments inhibit translation initiation. Mol Cell 43:613–623

13. Ivanov P, O'Day E, Emara MM, Wagner G, Lieberman J et al (2014) G-quadruplex structures contribute to the neuroprotective effects of angiogenin-induced tRNA fragments. Proc Natl Acad Sci U S A 111:18201–18206

Chapter 11

Isolation of Plasma Lipoproteins as a Source of Extracellular RNA

Kang Li, David K. Wong, Fu Sang Luk, Roy Y. Kim, and Robert L. Raffai

Abstract

Plasma lipoproteins are essential vehicles of lipid distribution for cellular energy and structural requirements as well as for excretion of lipid excess. Imbalances in lipoprotein metabolism are known to contribute to metabolic diseases ranging from vascular inflammation and atherosclerosis to obesity and diabetes. The lipid and protein cargo carried by lipoprotein subclasses have long been the focus of studies exploring the contribution of plasma lipoproteins in health and in metabolic disorders. More recent studies have revealed the presence of noncoding RNA as a new form of cargo carried by plasma lipoproteins. Lipoprotein-associated microRNAs have been identified to distribute differentially among plasma lipoprotein subclasses and contribute to cellular signaling. These findings highlight plasma lipoprotein-associated RNA as a potential source of biological signaling and warrant a renewed interest in the study of plasma lipoprotein biology. This chapter describes principles and methods based on density ultracentrifugation and size exclusion chromatography for the isolation of plasma lipoproteins as a source of extracellular RNA.

Key words Lipoprotein, Sequential density ultracentrifugation, FPLC chromatography, HDL, VLDL, LDL, Extracellular RNA

1 Introduction

Plasma lipoproteins have long been recognized for their essential role in distributing both energy-rich and structural lipids, as well as vitamins and micronutrients to cells throughout the mammalian organism [1]. Select lipoprotein classes, including chylomicrons and very-low density lipoproteins (VLDL) that are secreted by the intestine and liver, respectively, serve as the major mediators of lipid and micronutrient distribution (Fig. 1). Through catabolic and lipolytic processes that occur in the circulation and the endothelial lining of organs and tissues, such lipoproteins are converted to remnants including low-density lipoproteins (LDL) that are cleared by the liver [1]. An accumulation of remnant lipoproteins in plasma, caused by metabolic defects including through mutations in the low-density lipoprotein receptor, has been identified as an important source of systemic and vascular inflammation and atherosclerosis [2].

Tushar Patel (ed.), *Extracellular RNA: Methods and Protocols*, Methods in Molecular Biology, vol. 1740,
https://doi.org/10.1007/978-1-4939-7652-2_11, © Springer Science+Business Media, LLC 2018

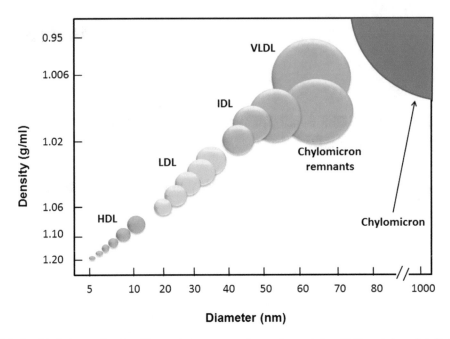

Fig. 1 Relationship between the densities and size among plasma lipoproteins. *VLDL* very low-density lipoprotein, *LDL* low-density lipoprotein, *HDL* high-density lipoprotein

An important cause of such lipoprotein-induced inflammation and cardiovascular disease has been linked to their uncontrolled absorption by monocytes in the circulation and macrophages in the vessel wall [3]. In contrast, high-density lipoproteins (HDL) that are derived primarily through the lipolytic remodeling of VLDL and chylomicrons have been shown to participate in the removal of cholesterol and lipid deposits from lesional macrophages which they deliver to the liver for excretion into bile in a process referred to a reverse cholesterol transport [4]. Such "cholesterol-efflux" property of HDL has long been touted as a primary mode of action in preventing atherosclerosis buildup and cardiovascular disease [5].

Beyond its role in mediating the cellular release of cholesterol, HDL is recognized to prevent cardiovascular diseases by exerting numerous anti-inflammatory properties [6]. Among these include the capacity for HDL to carry bioactive protein cargo such as the antioxidant enzyme paraoxonase that prevents the oxidation of lipids in lipoproteins including LDL and thereby the propensity for foam cell formation in the vessel wall [6]. HDL is also recognized to carry bioactive lipid cargo such as sphingosine-1-phosphate that provides a panoply of protective signaling properties in the cardiovascular and immune systems [7, 8]. Recent findings have introduced noncoding RNA including microRNA as yet a new class of nucleic acid cargo carried by HDL and other plasma lipoproteins [9]. Interestingly, the levels of select microRNA in both HDL and LDL have been shown to alter during conditions of metabolic excess including hyperlipidemia [9]. Moreover, HDL-associated microRNAs have been shown to participate in cellular signaling within the cardiovascular system [10]. Such exciting findings have spurred a renewed interest in the isolation and study of plasma lipoproteins both as biomarkers for disease states and mediators of RNA bio-distribution and intercellular communication.

A robust and widely used method to isolate plasma lipoproteins, first reported in 1955 by Richard Havel and colleagues while at the National Institutes of Health in Bethesda [11], is based on sequential density ultracentrifugation (SD-UC) of plasma that is adjusted to well-defined densities using potassium bromide salt. Another procedure commonly used to separate plasma lipoproteins makes use of size exclusion chromatography, often with a fast-protein liquid chromatography (FPLC) system combined with columns filled with high-resolution stationary phases. While more rapid and convenient than sequential density ultracentrifugation, FPLC separation of plasma lipoproteins is used most often as an analytical approach for the assessment of plasma lipoprotein profiles in experimental murine models of lipoprotein metabolism [12]. Affinity chromatography using columns linked to monoclonal antibodies specific to select apolipoproteins provides yet another approach to selectively isolate plasma lipoprotein subclasses [13]. However, the use of low pH required to elute lipoproteins retained by the immuno-affinity column poses unknown risk for the loss of nucleic acids from the purified lipoprotein. Thus, sequential density ultracentrifugation remains by far the gold standard method for the isolation of well-defined lipoprotein classes in sufficient quantities to allow for subsequent in vitro or in vivo studies of lipoprotein function and RNA composition. Moreover, the availability of smaller desktop-sized ultracentrifuges and rotor systems allows for the isolation of lipoproteins from as little as 2 mL of plasma which facilitates the study of lipoprotein biology in genetically engineered mouse models of human diseases [14]. This chapter describes principles and methods for isolation and characterization of lipoprotein classes from blood plasma.

2   Materials

2.1   Sequential Gradient Ultracentrifugation

1. Potassium bromide (KBr) (Sigma).
2. Optima MAX-XP tabletop ultracentrifuge (Beckman Coulter).
3. TLA-100.3 rotor (Beckman Coulter).
4. Polypropylene Quick-Seal 3.5 mL tubes (Beckman Coulter).
5. CentriTube slicer (Beckman Coulter).
6. 1 mL slip-tip disposable syringe (BD Biosciences).
7. BD PrecisionGlide needle, 21 G × 1.5 in. (BD Biosciences).
8. Optima XPN 90 floor-model ultracentrifuge (Beckman Coulter).
9. Type 50.2 Ti rotor (Beckman Coulter).
10. Polypropylene 39 mL Quick-Seal tubes (Beckman Coulter).
11. Phosphate buffered saline, pH 7.4 with 1 mM EDTA.

2.2 FPLC Chromatography	1. Isocratic HPLC pump with a manual Rheodyne sample injector (Fisher Scientific).

1. Isocratic HPLC pump with a manual Rheodyne sample injector (Fisher Scientific).

2. Programmable 96-well fraction collector (Fisher Scientific).

3. Superose 6, 10/300 GL FPLC size exclusion column (GE Healthcare).

2.3 SDS-PAGE and Coomassie Blue Detection

1. PROTEAN II xi cell (Bio-Rad).

2. 30% Acrylamide/Bis solution (Bio-Rad).

3. Ammonium persulfate (APS) (Bio-Rad).

4. TEMED (Bio-Rad).

5. ImageQuant LAS 4000.

2.4 Lipoprotein Cholesterol Analysis

1. Wako cholesterol E assay (Wako Diagnostics).

2. Control serum I (Wako Diagnostics).

3. Control serum II (Wako Diagnostics).

4. Microplate spectrophotometer (Thermo Fisher Scientific or any other brand).

2.5 Lipoprotein RNA Analysis

1. mirVana™ PARIS™ RNA and Native Protein Purification Kit (Thermo Fisher Scientific).

2. Sodium acetate, 3M, PH5.2 (Amresco LLC).

3. Ethanol, molecular biology grade (Sigma).

4. Agilent 2100 bioanalyzer instrument.

5. Agilent RNA 6000 pico kit.

6. Agilent small RNA kit.

3 Methods

3.1 Isolation of Very-Low and Low-Density Lipoprotein (VLDL/LDL) Fraction from Plasma

1. Collect blood from a human subject or from mice into EDTA coated tubes according to institutional guidelines. When bleeding mice for nonterminal experiments, one may typically obtain no more than 250 μL of blood from each mouse (*see* **Note 1**).

2. Spin the blood for 10 min at 2000 × g at 4 °C to remove erythrocytes and white cells.

3. Platelets must next be removed by spinning the plasma for 30 min at 15,000 × g.

4. Non-fasted plasma can sometimes produce a milky fat-rich layer of chylomicrons that can be removed by gentle pipetting if this class of lipoprotein is not of interest (*see* **Note 2**). Subsequently, gently pipette the clear platelet- and chylomicron-free supernatant.

5. Pool all the plasma into a fresh 15-mL tube kept on ice and record the exact volume.

6. Weigh out the needed amount of KBr (*see* **Note 3**) required to produce a density of 1.063 g/mL using the formula: plasma (mL) × 0.0834 = KBr (g). Add the KBr to the plasma and let the tube sit on ice then mix slowly using a wide bore pipet to avoid causing excessive shear stress in the solution.

7. Add 0.834 g KBr into 10 mL PBS to make d = 1.063 g/mL KBr/PBS solution.

8. Transfer the plasma to ultracentrifuge tubes using 3 mL syringes.

9. Add d = 1.063 g/mL KBr/PBS solution to fill the tube (total volume ~3.5 mL).

10. Balance the tubes; make sure that the weight difference between two tubes is within 0.1 g to avoid causing an imbalance in the rotor.

11. Seal the tubes with a preheated Beckman Tube Sealer.

12. Place the sealed ultracentrifuge tubes into a prechilled rotor (4 °C).

13. Place the rotor in the prechilled ultracentrifuge (4 °C), centrifuge at $100,000 \times g$.

14. After 24 h, stop the ultracentrifuge and gently take the tubes out of the rotor while avoiding disturbing the separated layers of lipoproteins.

15. Set up a Beckman Tube Slicer; rinse the blade and the holder with ddH$_2$O and allow it to dry.

16. Put in the blade and tighten the screw to secure the blade.

17. Place a tube into the tube holder and lower the holder arm using the bottom dial to secure the tube in place.

18. Adjust the cutting position in relation to the blade to cut approximately the top 1/5 of the tube (*see* **Note 4**) that will contain the VLDL/LDL (*see* **Note 5**).

19. Cut the tube in one movement of the slicer mechanism.

20. Insert a 21 gauge needle into the top portion of the tube above the blade in order to allow air entry during the subsequent aspiration step.

21. Insert a second needle attached to a 1 mL syringe immediately above the blade.

22. Gently aspirate the lipoprotein fraction by drawing on the syringe plunger.

23. Carefully disassemble the Tube Slicer instrument to allow for the removal of the top portion of the tube (*see* **Note 6**).

24. Slide the blade away from the tube and collect the infranatant in the bottom 4/5 portion of the tube that will contain the HDL (Fig. 2).

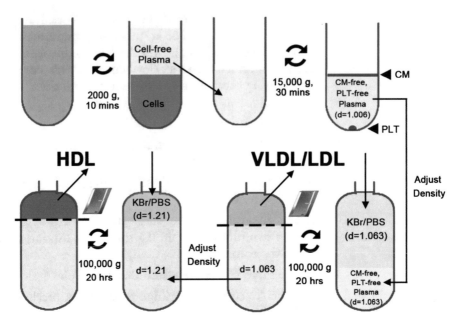

Fig. 2 Experimental workflow of sequential density ultracentrifugation (SD-UC) for lipoprotein fractionation (1). Collect and pool blood and centrifuge 2000 × g for 10 min to pellet blood cells; (2) Recover cell-free plasma and centrifuge 15,000 × g for 30 min to pellet platelets (PLT) and float chylomicrons (CM); (3) Collect PLT-free, CM-free plasma and add KBr to adjust its density to 1.063 g/mL; transfer it into a ultracentrifugation tube and fill the tube with saline that has been adjusted to the same density; seal the tubes and centrifuge 100,000 × g for 20 h to float the VLDL and LDL; (4) Cut the top of the tube to recover VLDL/LDL and add KBr to adjust the density of the remaining liquid from 1.063 to 1.21 g/mL; transfer it to a fresh ultracentrifugation tube and fill the tube with saline (density = 1.21 g/mL); seal the tubes and centrifuge 100,000 × g for 18 h to float the HDL fraction; (5) cut the top of the tube to collect HDL

3.2 Isolation of HDL Fraction

1. Precisely record the volume extracted from the bottom portion of the centrifuge tube. Weigh out the required amount of KBr to produce a density of 1.21 g/mL in the plasma using the formula provided in Table 1: d = 1.063 plasma (mL) × 0.235 = KBr (g). Add the KBr to the plasma and place the tube on ice. Mix slowly using a wide bore pipet.

2. Prepare d = 1.21 g/mL KBr/PBS by adding 3.15 g of KBr to 10 mL PBS according to Table 1.

3. Transfer the plasma to an ultracentrifuge tube using 3 mL syringes.

4. Add sufficient amount of cold d = 1.21 g/mL KBr/PBS solution to fill the tube.

5. Balance the tubes; make sure that the difference between two tubes is within 0.1 g.

6. Seal the tube with a Beckman Tube Sealer.

7. Place the ultracentrifuge tubes into a prechilled rotor (4 °C).

Table 1
Conversion factors for density adjustment among plasma, PBS, VLDL, LDL, and HDL using Solid KBr

	Initial density (g/mL)	Final density (g/mL)	Conversion factor
Plasma ≫ VLDL/LDL	1.006	1.063	0.0834
PBS ≫ VLDL/LDL	1.006	1.063	0.0834
VLDL/LDL ≫ HDL	1.063	1.21	0.235
PBS ≫ HDL	1.006	1.21	0.315
Plasma ≫ VLDL	1.006	1.019	0.0185
VLDL ≫ LDL	1.019	1.063	0.0629

8. Place the rotor in the prechilled ultracentrifuge (4 °C), centrifuge at $100,000 \times g$ for 24 h.

9. Remove the tubes while being careful not to disturb the lipoprotein layers.

10. Set up Beckman tube slicer as above making sure to cut at the 1/5 top portion of the tube.

11. Cut the tubes in one movement.

12. Aspirate the HDL fraction using a 1 mL syringe as detailed above, rinse the top of centrifuge tube.

13. Discard the infranatant.

3.3 Dialysis

1. Label dialysis cassette and make a dot in the corner that will be used for injection.

2. Equilibrate cassette 10 min in 2 L cold PBS.

3. Inject lipoprotein fraction into the cassette while taking care not to perforate the membrane.

4. Vacuum aspirate the residual air to ensure an efficient dialysis.

5. Dialyze in a cold room against PBS for 2 h and change the buffer using fresh PBS; subsequently, after a second 2 h period of dialysis, dialyze against fresh PBS overnight.

6. Remove the lipoprotein fractions from the dialysis cassettes using a 21 gauge needle and 1 mL syringe, and store on ice or in a refrigerator.

3.4 Sub-Fractionation of SD-UC-Isolated Plasma Lipoproteins by FPLC

1. Lipoprotein classes isolated by SD-UC can be further resolved by using size exclusion FPLC chromatography using a Superose 6, 10/300 GL column from GE Healthcare. A 200 μL volume of freshly isolated HDL or VLDL/LDL lipoprotein fraction is loaded into a 200 μL loop fixed onto a manual Rheodyne injector system that is in line with an isocratic HPLC pump set at a flow rate of 0.4 mL/min using PBS-EDTA as a mobile phase.

2. Upon injecting the loaded lipoproteins into the system, immediately start the fraction collector that is set to collect for 90 s for a total volume of 500 μL into a 96-well collection plate.

3. Maintain collection for at least 60 min after which the system is ready for a second injection.

4. Clean and store column according to guidelines provided by the manufacturer.

5. Determine the lipoprotein cholesterol distribution in the fractions using the Cholesterol E detection kit described below.

3.5 Determination of Cholesterol Levels in Lipoprotein Fractions

1. Prepare a standard curve provided in the Cholesterol E kit.

2. Prepare a 100-fold dilution of plasma samples and lipoprotein fractions using ddH_2O; vortex and keep on ice.

3. Add 100 μL diluted plasma, lipoprotein fractions and standards in triplicate to appropriate wells of a 96-well plate.

4. Add 150 μL cholesterol E buffer to appropriate wells in a 96-well plate.

5. Shake plate using a plate mixer and incubate at 37 °C for 5–15 min.

6. Read absorbance using a plate reader set at 690 nm and integrate data (Fig. 3).

3.6 Apolipoprotein Detection by SDS-PAGE

1. Mix a 100 μL volume of each of the lipoprotein fractions with Laemmli buffer. Heat the mixed samples at 95 °C for 5 min.

2. Using a gradient maker system, prepare 5–12% gradient polyacrylamide gels containing SDS as a denaturant (*see* **Note 7**).

3. Load the gels with a molecular-weight marker spanning 10–250 kDa along with the denatured lipoprotein samples and resolve the proteins by electrophoresis.

4. Visualization of resolved proteins in the PAGE is achieved by incubating the gel with Coomassie blue stain for 2 h.

5. Subsequently, the gels are destained in 5% methanol and 7.5% glacial acetic acid solution (*see* **Note 8)** and images are captured using an ImageQuant LAS 4000.

3.7 Lipoprotein RNA Extraction Using mirVana PARIS Kit

1. Add 400 μL VLDL/LDL or HDL samples in 2 mL tubes.

2. Add 400 μL pre-warmed 2× Denaturing Solution. Immediately mix thoroughly.

3. Add 800 μL Acid-Phenol:Chloroform, be sure to withdraw the bottom phase.

4. Vortex for 30–60 s to mix.

5. Centrifuge for 5 min at 14,000 × g at room temp to separate the mixture into aqueous and organic phases.

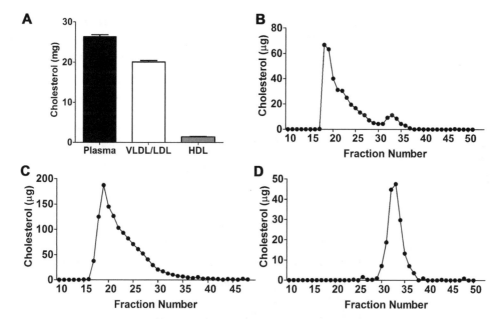

Fig. 3 Cholesterol profiles of total plasma and plasma lipoproteins separated by SD-UC and FPLC. VLDL/LDL and HDL were separated from plasma (6 mL) by sequential density ultracentrifugation. (a) The cholesterol content before and after isolation were determined; (b) Cholesterol profiles of total FPLC-fractionated plasma (200 µL), (c) VLDL/LDL (100 µL), (d) and HDL (75 µL)

6. Carefully remove the aqueous (upper) phase without disturbing the lower phase or the interphase, and transfer it to a fresh tube.

7. Add 1.25 volumes of 100% ethanol to the aqueous phase and mix thoroughly.

8. For each sample, place a filter cartridge into one of the collection tubes.

9. Pipet the lysate/ethanol mixture onto the filter cartridge. Apply a maximum of 700 µL to a filter cartridge at a time.

10. Centrifuge at $10,000 \times g$ for ~30 s.

11. Discard the flow-through, and repeat until all of the lysate/ethanol mixture is through the filter. Save the collection tube for the washing steps.

12. Apply 700 µL miRNA Wash Solution 1 to the filter cartridge and centrifuge at $10,000 \times g$ for ~15 s, discard the flow-through from the collection tube, and replace the filter cartridge into the same collection tube.

13. Apply 500 µL Wash Solution 2/3 and draw it through the filter cartridge as in the previous step.

14. Repeat with a second 500 µL of Wash Solution 2/3.

15. After discarding the flow-through from the last wash, replace the filter cartridge in the same collection tube and spin the assembly for 1 min at $10,000 \times g$ for 15 s, to remove residual fluid from the filter.

16. Transfer the filter cartridge into a fresh collection tube. Apply 50 µL of preheated (95 °C) nuclease-free water to the center of the filter, and close the cap. Centrifuge for ~30 s at 10,000 × g to recover the RNA.

17. Collect the eluate and store it at −80 °C.

3.8 RNA Concentration by Ethanol Precipitation

1. Combine all eluates from the same lipoprotein sample and add nuclease-free water to reach a final volume of 400 µL.

2. Add 50 µL 3 M PH 5.2 sodium acetate and −20 °C prechilled 100% ethanol (975 µL).

3. Incubate 30 min or overnight at −20 °C.

4. Centrifuge at 15,000 × g on a benchtop microcentrifuge at 30 min at 4 °C.

5. Remove and discard the supernatant. Leave the pellet intact.

6. Wash the pellet with 500 µL 70% ethanol at room temperature.

7. Centrifuge at 15,000 × g for 5 min.

8. Remove and discard the supernatant. Leave the pellet intact.

9. With the lid open, place the tube in a 37 °C heat block until the pellet is dry.

10. Add 10 µL nuclease-free water to dissolve the RNA pellet.

3.9 Lipoprotein Total RNA Characterization

11. Using an Agilent 2100 Bioanalyzer system, prepare a Gel-Dye mix by mixing 1 µL RNA dye concentrate with 65 µL filtered gel, vortex solution well, and spin the tube at 13,000 × g for 10 min at room temperature.

12. Load 9 µL Gel-Dye mix to appropriate well and prime the RNA Pico chip.

13. Load 9 µL Gel-Dye mix and the RNA conditioning solution to appropriate well.

14. Pipet 5 µL of RNA marker in the well for ladder and all 11 sample wells.

15. Pipet 1 µL of the heat denatured ladder into the ladder well.

16. Pipet 1 µL of sample in each of the 11 sample wells.

17. Vortex for 1 min at 2400 rpm in the IKA station.

18. Run the chip in the Agilent 2100 Bioanalyzer within 5 min.

3.10 Lipoprotein Small RNA Characterization

1. Prepare the Gel-Dye mixture by combining the RNA dye concentrate with filtered gel, vortex the solution well, and spin the tube at 13,000 × g for 10 min at room temperature.

2. Load 9 µL Gel-Dye mix to appropriate well and prime the small RNA chip.

3. Load 9 μL Gel-Dye mix and the RNA conditioning solution to appropriate wells.

4. Pipet 5 μL of RNA marker in the well for ladder and all 11 sample wells.

5. Pipet 1 μL of the heat denatured ladder into the ladder well.

6. Pipet 1 μL of sample in each of the 11 sample wells.

7. Vortex for 1 min at 2400 rpm in the IKA station.

8. Run the chip in the Agilent 2100 Bioanalyzer within 5 min.

4   Notes

1. Based on our experience in isolating RNA from plasma lipoprotein subclasses for subsequent biochemical and sequencing analysis, we highly recommend using a minimum volume of 5 mL of plasma. Indeed, our preparations of lipoprotein classes obtained from such a volume of fresh or frozen plasma have led to successful unbiased RNA sequencing experiments (Dr. David Erle, UCSF, unpublished data). However, unpublished data from our group also suggests that freezing plasma could alter the abundance of microRNA species in select lipoprotein classes. Thus one should take caution when designing a study aimed at examining RNA species with archived frozen plasma samples.

    A volume of 5 mL of plasma can be conveniently divided into two 3.5 mL centrifuge tubes to allow for rotor balancing during centrifugation in a tabletop ultracentrifuge. Alternatively, the entire 5 mL volume or even a larger volume of plasma can be loaded into large ultracentrifugation tubes (e.g., 39 mL Quick-Seal tubes) and a corresponding floor-model ultracentrifuge / rotor system (e.g., Optima XPN 90/ 50.2 Ti). Although 5 mL of plasma can be readily obtained from a human blood donor, it will be more challenging to derive from mice. Therefore when planning to isolate RNA from mouse lipoproteins it is advised that a minimum of 10–15 mice be used for a terminal bleeding. Larger cohorts of mice should be used in situations when the mice are to be maintained for further study as only smaller volumes of blood can be obtained under such circumstances.

2. Because of their high catabolic rate we recommend to avoid the isolation of chylomicrons together with the more stable VLDL/LDL fraction. The very high levels of neutral lipid associated with chylomicrons, especially in non-fasted plasma specimens, could also pose unknown problems and even a bias in RNA extraction/recovery that could be caused by excessive amounts of neutral lipid and foreign RNA possibly derived

from dietary sources [15]. We have found that gently pipetting any white layer that forms at the top of the plasma that is spun at $13,000 \times g$ for the removal of platelets generally results in the elimination of the chylomicron fraction. However, ultracentrifugation of virgin plasma overnight at $100,000 \times g$ will ensure the flotation of all chylomicrons to the top of the tube where they can be cut away from other lipoprotein subclasses and subsequently discarded or used as a source of RNA if so desired.

3. Potassium bromide salt (KBr) is highly hygroscopic and should be kept in a dry and preferably desiccant environment to prevent its hydration that would compromise its use to produce accurate density solutions. Because of this issue, it is recommended to make use of a densitometer to verify the density of the KBr-plasma samples as well as the KBr/PBS standard solutions.

4. The decision to cut the top 1/5 of the centrifuge tube after an overnight centrifugation of plasma is based on our experience in determining that this site is generally free of lipoproteins. The desired lipoproteins of lower density are known to float and accumulate in the top of the tube, while the lipoproteins of higher density sink to a lower portion of the tube.

5. Should there be a desire to separate VLDL from LDL, the density of the first centrifugation should be adjusted to $d = 1.019$ g/mL that will allow VLDL to float and LDL will sediment along with HDL in the infranatant. Subsequently, LDL can be separated from HDL by adjusting the infranatant to a density of 1.063 g/mL. Table 1 presents the factors required to calculate the adjustments of densities using KBr.

6. We have observed that lipoproteins will float to the very top of the tubes. To avoid possible losses of lipoproteins that may collect on the inside of the cap wall, it is important to rinse the top of the cut centrifuge tube using a portion of the liquid fraction that has been aspirated from the tube with a syringe.

7. The use of 5–12% gradient gels is essential in order to resolve the full spectrum of proteins associated with lipoproteins. The molecular weight of apoB-100 and apoB-48, two important structural components of low-density lipoproteins and chylomicron remnants, are approximately 550 and 210 kDa, respectively, and will resolve in the upper 25% of the gradient gel. Conversely, the size of apoE and apoA1 and all other apolipoproteins is less than 50 kDa and will resolve in the lower 50% of the gradient gel as illustrated in Fig. 4.

8. Destaining of a Coomassie blue gel can be assisted by introducing a few pieces of KimWipe paper that will absorb the blue dye released from the gel and will aid in clarifying the protein-negative portions of the gel (Fig. 5).

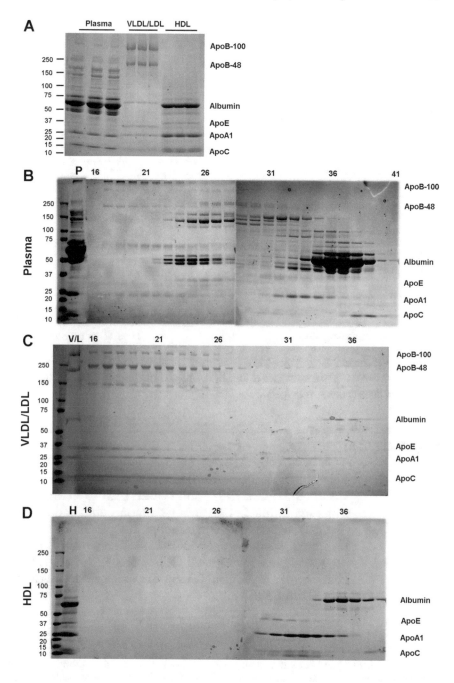

Fig. 4 Apolipoprotein distribution of total plasma and plasma lipoproteins separated by SD-UC and FPLC. VLDL/LDL and HDL were separated from plasma (6 mL) by sequential density ultracentrifugation. (**a**) SDS-PAGE analysis of total plasma (3 μL), VLDL/LDL (10 μL), and HDL (10 μL). (**b**, **c**, and **d**) SDS-PAGE analysis of FPLC fractions of 200 μL plasma (**b**), 100 μL VLDL/LDL (**c**), and 75 μL HDL (**d**). For each fraction, 90 μL sample was loaded. *P* plasma, *V/L* VLDL/LDL, *H* HDL

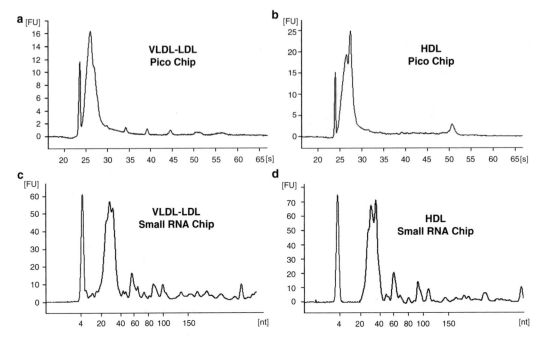

Fig. 5 Lipoprotein RNA Characterization by Agilent Bioanalyzer. Representative images of Agilent RNA 6000 Pico chip (**a, b**) and Small RNA chip (**c, d**) assays of total RNA isolated from plasma VLDL/LDL and HDL fractions isolated by sequential density ultracentrifugation

Acknowledgments

This work was supported by grants from the National Institutes of Health; 5U19CA179512 and 1U01HL126493 Extracellular RNA Communication Consortium Common Fund, and HL133575 to (R.L.R.) which was administered by the Northern California Institute for Research and Education. The work was performed at the Veterans Affairs Medical Center, San Francisco, CA. We thank Phat Duong and Allen Chung for excellent technical assistance with SDS-PAGE.

References

1. Havel RJ, Kane JP (2001) Introduction: structure and metabolism of plasma lipoproteins. In: Scriver CR, Beaudet AL, Sly WS, Valle D, Childs B, Kinzler KW, Vogelstein B (eds) The metabolic and molecular bases of inherited disease. McGraw-Hill, New York, pp 2705–2716

2. Mahley RW, Huang Y, Rall SC Jr (1999) Pathogenesis of type III hyperlipoproteinemia (dysbetalipoproteinemia): questions, quandaries, and paradoxes. J Lipid Res 40:1933–1949

3. Swirski FK, Libby P, Aikawa E, Alcaide P, Luscinskas FW, Weissleder R, Pittet MJ

(2007) Ly-6Chi monocytes dominate hypercholesterolemia-associated monocytosis and give rise to macrophages in atheromata. J Clin Invest 117:195–205

4. Tall AR, Yvan-Charvet L, Terasaka N, Pagler T, Wang N (2008) HDL, ABC transporters, and cholesterol efflux: implications for the treatment of atherosclerosis. Cell Metab 7:365–375

5. Murphy AJ, Westerterp M, Yvan-Charvet L, Tall AR (2012) Anti-atherogenic mechanisms of high density lipoprotein: effects on myeloid cells. Biochim Biophys Acta 1821:513–521

6. Barter PJ, Nicholls S, Rye KA, Anantharamaiah GM, Navab M, Fogelman AM (2004) Antiinflammatory properties of HDL. Circ Res 95:764–772

7. Nofer J-R, van der Giet M, Tölle M, Wolinska I, von Wnuck Lipinski K, Baba HA, Tietge UJ, Gödecke A, Ishii I, Kleuser B et al (2004) HDL induces NO-dependent vasorelaxation via the lysophospholipid receptor S1P₃. J Clin Invest 113:569–581

8. Tao R, Hoover HE, Honbo N, Kalinowski M, Alano CC, Karliner JS, Raffai R (2010) High-density lipoprotein determines adult mouse cardiomyocyte fate after hypoxia-reoxygenation through lipoprotein-associated sphingosine 1-phosphate. Am J Physiol Heart Circ Physiol 298:H1022–H1028

9. Vickers KC, Palmisano BT, Shoucri BM, Shamburek RD, Remaley AT (2011) MicroRNAs are transported in plasma and delivered to recipient cells by high-density lipoproteins. Nat Cell Biol 13:423–433

10. Tabet F, Vickers KC, Cuesta Torres LF, Wiese CB, Shoucri BM, Lambert G, Catherinet C, Prado-Lourenco L, Levin MG, Thacker S et al (2014) HDL-transferred microRNA-223 regulates ICAM-1 expression in endothelial cells. Nat Commun 5:3292

11. Havel RJ, Eder HA, Bragdon JH (1955) The distribution and chemical composition of ultra-centrifugally separated lipoproteins in human serum. J Clin Invest 34:1345–1353

12. Gaudreault N, Kumar N, Posada JM, Stephens KB, Reyes de Mochel NS, Eberle D, Olivas VR, Kim RY, Harms MJ, Johnson S et al (2012) ApoE suppresses atherosclerosis by reducing lipid accumulation in circulating monocytes and the expression of inflammatory molecules on monocytes and vascular endothelium. Arterioscler Thromb Vasc Biol 32:264–272

13. Raffaï R, Maurice R, Weisgraber K, Innerarity T, Wang X, MacKenzie R, Hirama T, Watson D, Rassart E, Milne R (1995) Molecular characterization of two monoclonal antibodies specific for the LDL receptor-binding site of human apolipoprotein E. J Lipid Res 36:1905–1918

14. Eberle D, Luk FS, Kim RY, Olivas VR, Kumar N, Posada JM, Li K, Gaudreault N, Rapp JH, Raffai RL (2013) Inducible Apoe gene repair in hypomorphic ApoE mice deficient in the low-density lipoprotein receptor promotes atheroma stabilization with a human-like lipoprotein profile. Arterioscler Thromb Vasc Biol 33:1759–1767

15. Baier SR, Nguyen C, Xie F, Wood JR, Zempleni J (2014) MicroRNAs are absorbed in biologically meaningful amounts from nutritionally relevant doses of cow milk and affect gene expression in peripheral blood mononuclear cells, HEK-293 kidney cell cultures, and mouse livers. J Nutr 144:1495–1500

Chapter 12

Droplet Digital PCR for Quantitation of Extracellular RNA

Irene K. Yan, Rishabh Lohray, and Tushar Patel

Abstract

Cell-to-cell communication involves the release of biological molecules into the extracellular space and their uptake by recipient cells. These molecules include RNA that can modulate cellular signaling and biological processes. To study extracellular RNA, highly sensitive and precise methods for their detection are needed. Digital polymerase chain reaction (dPCR) can be a useful method for detecting and analyzing extracellular RNA. The sensitivity of digital PCR can exceed that of quantitative PCR for low abundance targets such as extracellular RNA.

Key words Digital PCR, Extracellular RNA

1 Introduction

Digital polymerase chain reaction (PCR) is an emerging technique for the quantitation of nucleic acids [1]. The use of digital PCR for the measurement of extracellular RNA enables the measurement of small differences and thereby provides a greater sensitivity for the detection of rare transcripts. The use of digital PCR thus allows for more accurate determination of extracellular RNA in in vitro studies, as well as for diagnostic assays. Digital PCR involves the partitioning of a sample into tens of thousands of separate reactions. The reaction undergoes PCR either in real time or as an endpoint where each separate reaction will contain some or no copies of the gene of interest, and are separately analyzed. The number of reaction partitions that contain an amplified product is then counted. Digital PCR provides high precision, sensitivity, reproducibility, and dynamic range for the measurement of extracellular RNA [2]. In addition to the absolute quantification, the method can be used for analysis of other nucleic acids, gene copy number variation, rare event detection, and single cell analysis [3–6]. The sensitivity of digital PCR exceeds that of quantitative PCR for low abundance targets [5].

Tushar Patel (ed.), *Extracellular RNA: Methods and Protocols*, Methods in Molecular Biology, vol. 1740, https://doi.org/10.1007/978-1-4939-7652-2_12, © Springer Science+Business Media, LLC 2018

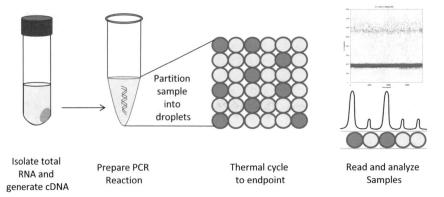

Fig. 1 Schematic overview of extracellular RNA detection by droplet digital PCR. Extracellular RNA is isolated from biological materials and cDNA generated. Samples are partitioned into thousands of droplets and subjected to endpoint PCR. Fluorescence is measured in each droplet and quantitated to obtain a measure of transcript present

Herein, we describe the use of droplet digital PCR (Fig. 1). In this technique, the reaction volume is generated in the form of a water-in-oil emulsion droplet, an endpoint PCR is performed using fluorescence-based detection technology, and individual droplet reactions are analyzed using a fluorescent detector [6]. Positive droplets are counted and a Poisson correction is applied to derive the mean number of target sequences within each droplet and used to estimate the average target concentration. Other approaches to digital PCR involve the use of fixed-volume chip-based partitioning that entail the use of different instruments and methods.

2   Materials

2.1   Equipment and Software

1. Thermal cycler. This will be used for cDNA synthesis and for ddPCR amplification.

2. Heat sealer. This is for foil sealing the sample plate prior to amplification.

3. Droplet generator (Bio-Rad, 186-4003). The QX200 Droplet Generator uses oil-based reagents and microfluidics mechanism to partition a single PCR reaction into 20,000 nanoliter-sized droplets.

4. Droplet Reader (Bio-Rad, 186-4002). The QX200 droplet reader is an automated sampler that analyzes each individual droplet using a two color detection system. The droplet reader uses a droplet reader plate holder and droplet reader oil (Bio-Rad).

5. Quantasoft Software. This will be used for data analysis.

2.2   cDNA Synthesis

1. Extracellular RNA. Total RNA should be used for this protocol. RNA should be DNase treated to prevent genomic DNA contamination. Concentration and purity of RNA should be validated for quality assessment.

2. cDNA synthesis kit. The QX200 is an open platform and iScript cDNA Synthesis Kit (Bio-Rad), or an alternative cDNA synthesis kit can be used for this assay.

2.3   ddPCR Reaction Setup

1. ddPCR master mix. The QX200 can use Taqman assays or EvaGreen chemistry and custom primers.

2. For Taqman-based assays, use Bio-Rad, 186-3005. Prepare the reaction master mix: 20 µl of master mix will contain 5 µl nuclease free water, 10 µl ddPCR Mastermix for Taqman FAM/VIC probes, 1 µl of ddPCR assay mix (20×), and 4 µl of template cDNA. Plate samples into a 96-well PCR plate in preparation for droplet generation. A multichannel pipette can then be used to load the samples into the Droplet Generator cartridge (*see* **Note 1**).

3. For EvaGreen, use Bio-Rad 186-4005. Prepare the reaction master mix: 20 µl of master mix will contain 4 µl nuclease free water, 2 µl Primer Pairs 5 µM, 10 µl of ddPCR master mix for Evagreen, and 4 µl of template cDNA.

4. cDNA template. cDNA concentration should be diluted to avoid saturation of target copy number. Serial dilutions should be used initially to determine expected ddPCR range.

5. Primers. When designing primers, follow same guidelines as qRT-PCR primers (*see* **Note 2**). Primer concentration should be 900 nM each, but can be adjusted based on assay.

6. Probe. The QX200 Droplet Digital PCR system is compatible with FAM dye and HEX or VIC secondary. Taqman assay probes or EvaGreen dsDNA binding dye chemistries can be used for detection (*see* **Note 3**). Probe concentration should be 250 nM but can be adjusted based on assay.

7. 96-well PCR plate for sample preparation.

2.4   Generation of Droplets

1. Droplet generator oil. There is separate oil depending on the probe-based or EvaGreen-based chemistries (*see* **Note 4**). For Taqman-based assays, use Bio-Rad, 186-3005, and for EvaGreen, use Bio-Rad 186-4005.

2. DG80 Cartridge (Bio-Rad, 186-4008). These cartridges hold eight samples each.

3. DG Gasket (Bio-Rad, 186-3009).

4. Cartridge Holder (Bio-Rad, 186-3051).

5. ddPCR Supermix. For Taqman-based assays, use the supermix for probes (Bio-Rad, 186-3023). For EvaGreen assays, use

EvaGreen supermix (Bio-Rad, 186-4034 and custom primers).

6. Multichannel pipettes. To manage samples efficiently, a p20 and p200 multichannel pipette is required.

7. Reagent trough. The samples are easiest to distribute using a reagent trough.

8. Pierceable Foil Heat Seat (Bio-Rad, 181-4040).

9. Eppendorf twin.tec 96-well plates, semi-skirted (Fisher, 951020346).

10. Plate sealer. A plate sealer is required to foil-seal the plate prior to PCR (*see* **Note 5**).

3   Methods

Prepare all reactions using nuclease free water and filtered pipette tips in a RNase-free work area.

3.1   cDNA Preparation

1. Prepare a minimum of 20 ng of DNase-treated RNA in 10 μl of nuclease free water. Manufacturer recommends RNA template 100 fg to 1 μg total RNA.

2. Mix 4 μl 5× iScript Buffer, 1 μl iScript RT, 0.2 μl RNase inhibitor (20 units/μl), and 4.8 μl water in PCR tubes. Add 10 μl RNA from previous step.

3. Incubate using the following reaction protocol: 5 min at 25 °C, 30 min at 42 °C, 5 min at 85 °C, and hold at 4 °C.

4. Template cDNA should be diluted such that it will not be saturating the droplet reader (*see* **Note 6**).

3.2   ddPCR Reaction Setup

1. Prepare the reaction master mix with water, ddPCR Supermix, Taqman FAM/VIC probes, and cDNA. If the samples are prepared and arranged on a PCR plate, it can be loaded into the Droplet Generator cartridge using the multichannel pipette (*see* **Note 1**).

3.3   Droplet Generation

1. Place the DG80 cartridge into the cartridge holder and lock in to place.

2. Using a multichannel pipette, transfer 20 μl sample into the DG80 cartridge's middle wells (*see* **Note 7**).

3. Secure the DG Gasket over the holder.

4. Place assembled cartridge and holder into the droplet generator, press button to close door. Droplets will automatically generate.

5. After droplets are generated, remove the cartridge holder and carefully remove and discard the gasket.

6. Slowly transfer 35 µl of droplets into column of Eppendorf twin.tec 96-well plate (*see* **Note 8**).

7. Repeat **steps 3–7** until all samples are droplet generated and transferred to the 96-well plate.

8. Place foil seal on top of plate and depress hotplate for 5 s.

9. Rotate plate and depress hotplate again for 5 s (*see* **Note 9**).

3.4 PCR Amplification

1. Load sealed plate into thermocycler and close lid. Run the protocol for endpoint PCR outlined in Tables 1 or 2. Use a 2.5 °C/s ramp rate to ensure each droplet reaches proper temperature. Plate should be read immediately after or stored at 4 °C overnight.

3.5 Droplet Reading and Defining Experiment

1. Transfer 96-well plate into the droplet reader plate holder.

2. Place plate and holder into the QX200 droplet reader.

3. Set up the experiment in Quantasoft Software. Select experiment to define analysis.

4. Enter details for sample ID and target for each well.

Table 1
Taqman assay

Segment	Cycles	Temperature (°C)	Time (s)
1	1	95	600
2	40	94	30
		60	60
3	1	98	600

Table 2
EvaGreen assay

Segment	Cycles	Temperature (°C)	Time (s)
1	1	95	300
2	40	95	30
		60	60
3	1	4	300
	1	90	300

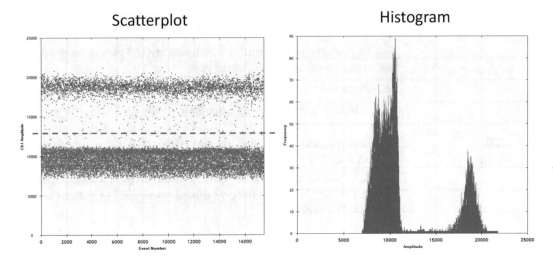

Fig. 2 Representative data from droplet digital PCR. Droplets with positive PCR product can be separated from those without on the scatter plot (*left*) or on the histogram (*right*). Optimization of protocol may be required to ensure adequate separation of positive droplets from negative droplets

5. Ensure there is appropriate droplet reader oil in the instrument and the waste compartment is emptied.

6. Select Run to begin data acquisition (*see* **Note 10**).

3.6 Data Analysis

1. After sample run is complete, software will automatically open the first well with data to begin analysis.

2. For absolute quantification analysis, automatic thresholding will determine target concentration based on positive and negative populations in fluorescence amplitude.

3. Thresholds can be manually adjusted on scatter plots or histograms for each sample or a set of samples. To determine the threshold setting, there should be a distinct positive and negative population (*see* **Note 11**) (Fig. 2).

4. The concentration is reported as copies/µl of the final ddPCR reaction (*see* **Note 12**).

4 Notes

1. It is best to prepare a little extra to make up for lost volume from pipetting. It is critical that you transfer exactly 20 µl into cartridge.

2. Primers validated for qRT-PCR should be used for ddPCR.

3. Probe sequence should be between the two primers of the amplicon and not overlap. The probe should be 3–10 °C higher than the primers, <30 nucleotides length, and should not have a G at the 5′ end.

4. Droplet generator oil has a limited shelf life and is important to use fresh oil or it can cause lower droplet counts.

5. The sealer should be warmed up approximately 15 min prior to use.

6. This will need to be optimized by the user and can be done by using different range of dilutions.

7. Make sure the tip reaches the bottom of the wells and avoid bubbles as this will affect the droplet counts.

8. It is critical that this is done slowly and uniformly to prevent shearing of droplets.

9. Confirm that all wells are sealed properly. Evaporation may occur and affect quantitation.

10. If the instrument has been idle for over 1 month, priming the system may be necessary to flush out reagents.

11. It is best to compare positive, negative, and unknown sample next to each other. Set the threshold for negative and apply the same threshold across all samples.

12. For more information about reporting results, follow the MIQE guidelines [7, 8].

Acknowledgments

This work was supported by the National Institutes of Health (USA) Office of the Director through grant UH3 TR000884. We acknowledge the expert assistance of Caitlyn Foerst and thank the members of our laboratories for their contributions.
Disclosures. None.

References

1. Morley AA (2014) Digital PCR: a brief history. Biomol Detect Quantif 1(1):1–2. https://doi.org/10.1016/j.bdq.2014.06.001

2. Bellingham SA, Shambrook M, Hill AF (2017) Quantitative analysis of exosomal miRNA via qPCR and digital PCR. Methods Mol Biol 1545:55–70. https://doi.org/10.1007/978-1-4939-6728-5_5

3. Yan IK, Wang X, Asmann YW, Haga H, Patel T (2016) Circulating extracellular RNA markers of liver regeneration. PLoS One 11(7):e0155888. https://doi.org/10.1371/journal.pone.0155888

4. Takahashi K, Yan IK, Kim C, Kim J, Patel T (2014) Analysis of extracellular RNA by digital PCR. Front Oncol 4:129. https://doi.org/10.3389/fonc.2014.00129

5. Taylor SC, Laperriere G, Germain H (2017) Droplet digital PCR versus qPCR for gene expression analysis with low abundant targets: from variable nonsense to publication quality data. Sci Rep 7(1):2409. https://doi.org/10.1038/s41598-017-02217-x

6. McDermott GP, Do D, Litterst CM, Maar D, Hindson CM, Steenblock ER, Legler TC, Jouvenot Y, Marrs SH, Bemis A, Shah P, Wong J, Wang S, Sally D, Javier L, Dinio T, Han C, Brackbill TP, Hodges SP, Ling Y, Klitgord N, Carman GJ, Berman JR, Koehler RT, Hiddessen AL, Walse P, Bousse L, Tzonev S, Hefner E, Hindson BJ, Cauly TH 3rd, Hamby K, Patel VP, Regan JF, Wyatt PW, Karlin-Neumann GA, Stumbo DP, Lowe AJ (2013) Multiplexed target detection using DNA-binding dye chemistry in droplet digital PCR. Anal Chem 85(23):11619–11627. https://doi.org/10.1021/ac403061n

7. Huggett JF, Foy CA, Benes V, Emslie K, Garson JA, Haynes R, Hellemans J, Kubista

M, Mueller RD, Nolan T, Pfaffl MW, Shipley GL, Vandesompele J, Wittwer CT, Bustin SA (2013) The digital MIQE guidelines: minimum information for publication of quantitative digital PCR experiments. Clin Chem 59(6):892–902.   https://doi.org/10.1373/clinchem.2013.206375

8. Huggett JF, Cowen S, Foy CA (2015) Considerations for digital PCR as an accurate molecular diagnostic tool. Clin Chem 61(1):79–88.   https://doi.org/10.1373/clinchem.2014.221366

Chapter 13

Preparation of Small RNA NGS Libraries from Biofluids

Alton Etheridge, Kai Wang, David Baxter, and David Galas

Abstract

Next generation sequencing (NGS) is a powerful method for transcriptome analysis. Unlike other gene expression profiling methods, such as microarrays, NGS provides additional information such as splicing variants, sequence polymorphisms, and novel transcripts. For this reason, NGS is well suited for comprehensive profiling of the wide range of extracellular RNAs (exRNAs) in biofluids. ExRNAs are of great interest because of their possible biological role in cell-to-cell communication and for their potential use as biomarkers or for therapeutic purposes. Here, we describe a modified protocol for preparation of small RNA libraries for NGS analysis. This protocol has been optimized for use with low-input exRNA-containing samples, such as plasma or serum, and has modifications designed to reduce the sequence-specific bias typically encountered with commercial small RNA library construction kits.

Key words miRNA, Extracellular RNA, Sequencing, Biofluid, Serum, Plasma

1 Introduction

Extracellular RNAs have been detected in nearly all human biofluids. While the biological role of exRNAs in biofluids remains largely unclear, they are of significant interest because of their potential use as biomarkers and for therapeutic purposes. NGS has been used extensively to characterize the spectrum of exRNAs in circulation. However, commercial small RNA library preparation kits are typically designed for samples containing higher concentrations of RNA than are available in most biofluid samples. Additionally, libraries made with many commercial small RNA library kits exhibit strong sequence-specific bias which has the indirect effect of reducing library complexity and can result in misleading and incomplete RNA profiles.

Key advantages of the small RNA library preparation protocol we describe here (Fig. 1) include the use of degenerate nucleotides on the ends of the 3′ and 5′ adapters, the use of high adapter concentrations, and increased amounts of polyethylene glycol (PEG) in the ligation steps. Adapters containing degenerate bases have been found to reduce the bias introduced during ligations [1–5],

Tushar Patel (ed.), *Extracellular RNA: Methods and Protocols*, Methods in Molecular Biology, vol. 1740,
https://doi.org/10.1007/978-1-4939-7652-2_13, © Springer Science+Business Media, LLC 2018

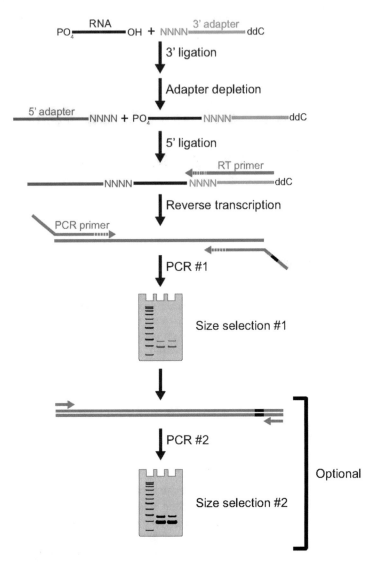

Fig. 1 Schematic of library construction workflow. Libraries are prepared by sequential ligation of adapters onto the 3′ and 5′ ends of the sample RNA. After the 3′ ligation, excess adapter is removed enzymatically before adding the 5′ adapter in order to reduce the amount of adapter dimer generated. Following the ligations, the sample is reverse transcribed with a primer complementary to the 3′ adapter. The libraries are amplified and indexed during the first PCR and size selected to enrich for the desired size range of RNA inserts and to remove adapter dimer side products. As an option, two rounds of PCR and size selection can be performed to further remove adapter dimer contamination in the library

leading to better representation of diverse sequences in the sample. Additionally, the use of high adapter concentrations and the macromolecular crowding agent, PEG, reduces bias by driving the ligation reactions towards completion. It should be noted, however, that the use of improved ligation conditions also results in the formation of more adapter dimers and other ligation side products, so careful purification of desired products away from unwanted products is critical for the success of this protocol. In some cases, two sequential amplification and gel purification steps can be required to effectively remove adapter dimers. Specific notes on these issues are included below.

2 Materials

2.1 Ligation—3′ Adapter

1. Dissolve 2.5 g of PEG 8000 in 10 mL of RNase-free water to make 25% PEG 8000 solution.

2. Aliquot 6 μL of 25% PEG 8000 into thin-walled 0.2 mL PCR tubes or strip tubes (*see* **Note 1**). Dry PEG completely in a vacuum concentrator at 37 °C. Dried PEG should appear as a flaky, white pellet in the bottom of each tube. Cap tubes and store desiccated at room temperature. After adding RNA and ligation reagents these tubes will yield a final PEG concentration of 15% for the 3′ ligation reaction (*see* **Note 2**).

3. Adenylated 3′ adapter oligo (sequence in Table 1) resuspended at 10 μM in 10 mM Tris–Cl pH 8. Freeze at −70 °C in small aliquots. Although we have found the 3′ adapter to be stable for multiple freeze-thaw cycles, it is best to aliquot in small volumes and minimize the number of times each aliquot is thawed.

4. T4 RNA ligase 2, truncated KQ (NEB) and supplied T4 RNA ligase reaction buffer (*see* **Note 3**).

5. RNaseOut RNAse inhibitor (Invitrogen).

2.2 Adapter Depletion (See Note 4)

1. Single-stranded DNA binding protein (SSBP; Promega) diluted to 1 μg/μL in 1× T4 RNA ligase reaction buffer just before use.

2. 5′ deadenylase (NEB).

3. RecJ exonuclease (NEB).

2.3 Ligation—5′ Adapter

1. 5′ adapter oligo (sequence in Table 1) resuspended at 25 μM in 1 mM sodium citrate pH 6.4. Freeze at −70 °C small aliquots.

2. T4 RNA ligase 1 (NEB).

3. 10 mM ATP. Make small aliquots and store at −20 °C. Aliquots are stable for several freeze-thaw cycles.

2.4 Reverse Transcription

1. Reverse transcription primer (RT primer; sequence in Table 1) resuspended at 10 μM in 10 mM Tris–Cl pH 8. Aliquot and store at −20 °C.

2. Superscript III reverse transcriptase with supplied 5× first strand reaction buffer and 100 mM DTT (Invitrogen).

Table 1
List of oligonucleotides

Name	Sequence (5′–3′)	Purification
3′ adapter	/5rApp/(N:25252525)(N)(N)(N)TGGÁAATTCTCGGGTGCCAAGG/3ddC/	HPLC
5′ adapter	rGrUrUrCrArGrArGrUrUrCrUrArCrArGrUrCrCrGrArGrArUrCr(N:25252525)r(N)r(N)r(N)	Desalted
RT primer	GCCTTGGCACCCGAGAATTCCA	Desalted
RP1	AATGATACGGCGACCACCGAGATCTACACGTTCAGAGTTCTACAGTCCGA	HPLC
RPI1	CAAGCAGAAGACGGCATACGAGATCGTGATGTGACTGGAGTTCCTTGGCACCCGAGAATTCCA	HPLC
RPI2	CAAGCAGAAGACGGCATACGAGATACATCGGTGACTGGAGTTCCTTGGCACCCGAGAATTCCA	HPLC
RPI3	CAAGCAGAAGACGGCATACGAGATGCCTAAGTGACTGGAGTTCCTTGGCACCCGAGAATTCCA	HPLC
RPI4	CAAGCAGAAGACGGCATACGAGATTGGTCAGTGACTGGAGTTCCTTGGCACCCGAGAATTCCA	HPLC
RPI5	CAAGCAGAAGACGGCATACGAGATCACTGTGTGACTGGAGTTCCTTGGCACCCGAGAATTCCA	HPLC
RPI6	CAAGCAGAAGACGGCATACGAGATATTGGCGTGACTGGAGTTCCTTGGCACCCGAGAATTCCA	HPLC
RPI7	CAAGCAGAAGACGGCATACGAGATGATCTGTGACTGGAGTTCCTTGGCACCCGAGAATTCCA	HPLC
RPI8	CAAGCAGAAGACGGCATACGAGATTCAAGTGTGACTGGAGTTCCTTGGCACCCGAGAATTCCA	HPLC
RPI9	CAAGCAGAAGACGGCATACGAGATCTGATCGTGACTGGAGTTCCTTGGCACCCGAGAATTCCA	HPLC
RPI10	CAAGCAGAAGACGGCATACGAGATAAGCTAGTGACTGGAGTTCCTTGGCACCCGAGAATTCCA	HPLC
RPI11	CAAGCAGAAGACGGCATACGAGATGTAGCCGTGACTGGAGTTCCTTGGCACCCGAGAATTCCA	HPLC
RPI12	CAAGCAGAAGACGGCATACGAGATTACAAGGTGACTGGAGTTCCTTGGCACCCGAGAATTCCA	HPLC
RPI13	CAAGCAGAAGACGGCATACGAGATTTGACTGTGACTGGAGTTCCTTGGCACCCGAGAATTCCA	HPLC
RPI14	CAAGCAGAAGACGGCATACGAGATGGAACTGTGACTGGAGTTCCTTGGCACCCGAGAATTCCA	HPLC
RPI15	CAAGCAGAAGACGGCATACGAGATTGACATGTGACTGGAGTTCCTTGGCACCCGAGAATTCCA	HPLC
RPI16	CAAGCAGAAGACGGCATACGAGATGGGTGACTGGAGTTCCTTGGCACCCGAGAATTCCA	HPLC

RPI17	CAAGCAGAAGACGGCATACGAGATCTCTACGTGACTGGAGTTCCTTGGCACCCGAGAATTCCA	HPLC
RPI18	CAAGCAGAAGACGGCATACGAGATGCGGACGTGACTGGAGTTCCTTGGCACCCGAGAATTCCA	HPLC
RPI19	CAAGCAGAAGACGGCATACGAGATTTCACGTGACTGGAGTTCCTTGGCACCCGAGAATTCCA	HPLC
RPI20	CAAGCAGAAGACGGCATACGAGATGGCCACGTGACTGGAGTTCCTTGGCACCCGAGAATTCCA	HPLC
RPI21	CAAGCAGAAGACGGCATACGAGATCGAAACGTGACTGGAGTTCCTTGGCACCCGAGAATTCCA	HPLC
RPI22	CAAGCAGAAGACGGCATACGAGATCGTACGGTGACTGGAGTTCCTTGGCACCCGAGAATTCCA	HPLC
RPI23	CAAGCAGAAGACGGCATACGAGATCCACTCGTGACTGGAGTTCCTTGGCACCCGAGAATTCCA	HPLC
RPI24	CAAGCAGAAGACGGCATACGAGATGCTACCGTGACTGGAGTTCCTTGGCACCCGAGAATTCCA	HPLC
RPI25	CAAGCAGAAGACGGCATACGAGATATCAGTGACTGGAGTTCCTTGGCACCCGAGAATTCCA	HPLC
RPI26	CAAGCAGAAGACGGCATACGAGATGCTCATGTGACTGGAGTTCCTTGGCACCCGAGAATTCCA	HPLC
RPI27	CAAGCAGAAGACGGCATACGAGATAGGAATGTGACTGGAGTTCCTTGGCACCCGAGAATTCCA	HPLC
RPI28	CAAGCAGAAGACGGCATACGAGATCTTTGGTGACTGGAGTTCCTTGGCACCCGAGAATTCCA	HPLC
RPI29	CAAGCAGAAGACGGCATACGAGATTAGTTGGTGACTGGAGTTCCTTGGCACCCGAGAATTCCA	HPLC
RPI30	CAAGCAGAAGACGGCATACGAGATCCGGTGGTGACTGGAGTTCCTTGGCACCCGAGAATTCCA	HPLC
RPI31	CAAGCAGAAGACGGCATACGAGATATCGTGGTGACTGGAGTTCCTTGGCACCCGAGAATTCCA	HPLC
RPI32	CAAGCAGAAGACGGCATACGAGATTGAGTGGTGACTGGAGTTCCTTGGCACCCGAGAATTCCA	HPLC
RPI33	CAAGCAGAAGACGGCATACGAGATCGCCTGGTGACTGGAGTTCCTTGGCACCCGAGAATTCCA	HPLC
RPI34	CAAGCAGAAGACGGCATACGAGATGCCATGGTGACTGGAGTTCCTTGGCACCCGAGAATTCCA	HPLC
RPI35	CAAGCAGAAGACGGCATACGAGATAAAATGGTGACTGGAGTTCCTTGGCACCCGAGAATTCCA	HPLC
RPI36	CAAGCAGAAGACGGCATACGAGATTGTTGGGTGACTGGAGTTCCTTGGCACCCGAGAATTCCA	HPLC

(continued)

Table 1
(continued)

Name	Sequence (5′–3′)	Purification
RPI37	CAAGCAGAAGACGGCATACGAGATATTCCGGTGACTGGAGTTCCTTGGCACCCGAGAATTCCA	HPLC
RPI38	CAAGCAGAAGACGGCATACGAGATAGCTAGGTGACTGGAGTTCCTTGGCACCCGAGAATTCCA	HPLC
RPI39	CAAGCAGAAGACGGCATACGAGATGTATAGGTGACTGGAGTTCCTTGGCACCCGAGAATTCCA	HPLC
RPI40	CAAGCAGAAGACGGCATACGAGATTCTGAGGTGACTGGAGTTCCTTGGCACCCGAGAATTCCA	HPLC
RPI41	CAAGCAGAAGACGGCATACGAGATGTCGTCGTGACTGGAGTTCCTTGGCACCCGAGAATTCCA	HPLC
RPI42	CAAGCAGAAGACGGCATACGAGATCGATTAGTGACTGGAGTTCCTTGGCACCCGAGAATTCCA	HPLC
RPI43	CAAGCAGAAGACGGCATACGAGATGCTGTAGTGACTGGAGTTCCTTGGCACCCGAGAATTCCA	HPLC
RPI44	CAAGCAGAAGACGGCATACGAGATATTATAGTGACTGGAGTTCCTTGGCACCCGAGAATTCCA	HPLC
RPI45	CAAGCAGAAGACGGCATACGAGATGAATGAGTGACTGGAGTTCCTTGGCACCCGAGAATTCCA	HPLC
RPI46	CAAGCAGAAGACGGCATACGAGATTCGGGAGTGACTGGAGTTCCTTGGCACCCGAGAATTCCA	HPLC
RPI47	CAAGCAGAAGACGGCATACGAGATCTTCGAGTGACTGGAGTTCCTTGGCACCCGAGAATTCCA	HPLC
RPI48	CAAGCAGAAGACGGCATACGAGATTGCCGAGTGACTGGAGTTCCTTGGCACCCGAGAATTCCA	HPLC
Universal forward primer	AATGATACGGCGACCACCGAG	Desalted
Universal reverse primer	CAAGCAGAAGACGGCATACGA	Desalted

Name, sequence, and purification of each oligonucleotide used in this protocol (*see* **Notes 19** and **20**)

3. RNaseOut RNAse inhibitor (Invitrogen).

4. 12.5 mM dNTP mix (*see* **Note 5**).

2.5 PCR Amplification and Size Selection 1

1. NEBNext Ultra II Q5 PCR master mix (NEB).

2. Forward PCR primer, RP1 (sequence in Table 1) resuspended at 20 µM.

3. Indexed reverse PCR primer RPI1–RPI48 (sequences in Table 1) resuspended at 20 µM.

4. DNA Clean and Concentrator 5 columns (Zymo Research) or AMPure XP magnetic beads (Beckman Coulter).

5. 3% agarose cassettes and supplied marker 30G for PippinHT (Sage Science).

2.6 PCR Amplification and Size Selection 2

1. KAPA 2× real-time PCR master mix (KAPA Biosystems).

2. Universal forward and universal reverse PCR primers (sequences in Table 1) resuspended and combined in a cocktail at 20 µM each (Universal PCR primer cocktail).

3. DNA Clean and Concentrator 5 columns (Zymo Research) or AMPure XP magnetic beads (Beckman Coulter).

4. 3% agarose cassettes and supplied marker 30G for PippinHT (Sage Science).

3 Methods

3.1 Ligation—3′ Adapter

1. Preheat thermal cycler to 70 °C.

2. Combine the following in a PCR tube containing dried PEG. The total volume added to the tube should be 6 µL.

RNA (*see* **Note 6**)	x µL
3′ adapter (10 µM)	1 µL
Water	To 6 µL

3. Incubate in thermal cycler at 70 °C for 2 min to denature sample, then immediately place tube on ice for at least 2 min.

4. Keeping the tube on ice, add the following reagents. The total volume will be 10 µL (*see* **Note 7**). Mix well and incubate the tube at 25 °C for 2 h (*see* **Notes 8–10**).

T4 RNA ligase reaction buffer	1 µL
RNaseOut	1 µL
T4 RNL2 KQ	1 µL

3.2 Adapter Depletion

1. Add 1 µL of SSBP (diluted to 1 µg/µL in 1× T4 RNA ligase reaction buffer) to each tube and incubate at 25 °C for 10 min.

2. Add 1 µL of 5′ deadenylase, mix, and incubate at 30 °C for 1 h.

3. Add 1 µL of RecJ, mix, and incubate at 37 °C for 1 h.

4. Transfer tube to ice.

3.3 Ligation—5′ Adapter

1. In a separate PCR tube, add 1 µL of 5′ adapter (25 µM) and denature by heating to 70 °C for 2 min. Immediately place tube on ice for 2 min (*see* **Note 11**).

2. On ice, add the following reagents to the tube of ligated, adapter-depleted RNA.

Denatured 5′ adapter	1 µL
ATP (10 mM)	1 µL
T4 RNA ligase 1	1 µL

3. Incubate the tube at 25 °C for 1 h.

3.4 Reverse Transcription

1. In a new PCR tube, combine the following. Heat to 70 °C for 2 min and immediately place the tube on ice (*see* **Note 12**).

Ligated RNA from previous step	6 µL
RT primer (10 µM)	1 µL

2. Add the following reagents to the tube of denatured RNA and RT primer and mix well. The total volume will be 12.5 µL.

5× first strand reaction buffer	2 µL
DTT (100 mM)	1 µL
dNTP mix (12.5 mM)	0.5 µL
RNaseOut	1 µL
Superscript III reverse transcriptase	1 µL

3. Incubate at 55 °C for 1 h followed by 70 °C for 15 min. Transfer tube to ice if proceeding immediately to PCR amplification. Alternatively, the cDNA may be stored at −20 °C before continuing to PCR amplification.

3.5 PCR Amplification and Size Selection 1 (See Note 13)

1. In a new PCR tube, combine the following reagents and mix well (*see* **Note 14**).

NEBNext Ultra II Q5 2× PCR master mix	25 µL
RP1 forward PCR primer (20 µM)	2 µL
RPI(1–48) reverse PCR primer (20 µM)	2 µL
cDNA from previous step	12.5 µL
Water	8.5 µL

2. Amplify the cDNA using the following program.

98 °C	30 s	Initial denaturation
98 °C	10 s	4 cycles
60 °C	30 s	
65 °C	30 s	
65 °C	2 min	Final extension

3. Purify the PCR product using a DNA Clean and Concentrator 5 column according to the manufacturer's protocol, and elute in 21 μL of elution buffer. Alternatively, if preparing several libraries at once, AMPure XP magnetic beads can be used for PCR cleanup. Add 100 μL of resuspended, room temperature AMPure XP beads to each 50 μL PCR reaction and mix well. Allow the tube to stand at room temperature for 5 min and then place on magnetic stand to collect beads (approximately 2 min). Remove supernatant and wash beads once with 150 μL of fresh 80% ethanol. Remove ethanol and allow beads to dry for 5 min. Bound material should be eluted from beads using 23 μL of 0.1× TE or water. Usually 21 μL can be recovered. Minimize bead carryover.

4. Prepare 3% agarose cassette for PippinHT. Add 5 μL of marker 30G to each sample and mix well (*see* **Note 15**).

5. Set PippinHT to select the range of 133–161 bp for miRNAs (*see* **Note 16**). Load samples and start the PippinHT run.

6. When run is complete, collect the eluate and concentrate in a vacuum concentrator until the volume is less than or equal to 22.5 μL.

3.6 PCR Amplification and Size Selection 2

1. Adjust the sample volume to 22.5 μL with water.

2. In a new PCR tube, combine the following reagents and mix well (*see* **Note 17**).

KAPA 2X real-time PCR master mix	25 μL
Universal PCR primer cocktail (20 μM)	2.5 μL
Purified PCR product from previous step	22.5 μL

3. Amplify the gel purified PCR product for additional 5–20 cycles until the fluorescent intensity of each sample is between the lowest and highest standards included with the PCR master mix using the following program.

98 °C	45 s	Initial denaturation
98 °C	15 s	5–20 cycles
60 °C	30 s	
72 °C	20 s	
72 °C	2 min	Final extension

4. Purify the PCR product using a DNA Clean and Concentrator 5 column according to the manufacturer's protocol, and elute in 21 µL of elution buffer. Alternatively, if preparing several libraries at once, AMPure XP magnetic beads can be used for PCR cleanup. Add 100 µL of resuspended, room temperature AMPure XP beads to each 50 µL PCR reaction and mix well. Allow the tube to stand at room temperature for 5 min and then place on magnetic stand to collect beads (approximately 2 min). Remove supernatant and wash beads once with 150 µL of fresh 80% ethanol. Remove ethanol and allow beads to dry for 5 min. Bound material should be eluted from beads using 23 µL of 0.1× TE or water. Usually 21 µL can be recovered. Minimize bead carryover.

5. Prepare 3% agarose cassette for PippinHT. Add 5 µL of marker 30G to each sample and mix well.

6. Set PippinHT to select the range of 133–161 bp for miRNAs (*see* **Note 16**). Load samples and start the PippinHT run.

7. When run is complete, collect the eluate and concentrate in a vacuum concentrator until the volume is approximately 10–15 µL. Load 1 µL on a DNA 1000 chip or high sensitivity DNA chip and run on a Bioanalyzer to check the library size (*see* **Note 18**).

4   Notes

1. 25% PEG is viscous. Care must be taken when aliquoting. Using a positive displacement pipette may be helpful.

2. Higher concentrations of PEG enhance ligation efficiency and lead to reduced sequence bias, but also increase the amount of adapter dimer formed, especially when the input RNA concentration is low. We have found a final concentration of 15% PEG in the 3′ ligation to be a good compromise between reduced bias and increased adapter dimer. However, the final PEG concentration can be adjusted between 10% and 25% depending on the amount of input RNA used.

3. T4 RNL2 KQ contains two mutations which make it preferable to other truncated T4 RNA ligase 2 variants. The K227Q mutation reduces side products and the R55K mutation

increases the rate of ligation compared to the K227Q mutant alone [6, 7].

4. Because of the degenerate bases at the ends of the 3′ and 5′ adapters, many methods used to prevent adapter dimer formation in commercial small RNA library construction kits are largely ineffective with these adapters. While enzymatic digestion of unligated 3′ adapter is more time consuming than other methods, we have found it to be the most effective way to prevent adapter dimer formation.

5. dNTP mix is supplied at 25 mM concentration. Dilute 1:2 and store in small aliquots at 12.5 mM.

6. This protocol has been used successfully with total RNA purified from 100 μL of serum, plasma and urine.

7. Although only 9 μL of reagents are added to the tube, the final volume of the 3′ ligation will be approximately 10 μL because of the volume of the PEG.

8. Higher concentrations of 3′ adapter reduce sequence bias, but also increase the amount of adapter dimer formed. For libraries made from RNA isolated from 100 μL of serum, plasma, and urine, we use 10 picomoles of 3′ adapter per ligation. The amount of 3′ adapter added to the ligation may be varied from 1 to 50 picomoles.

9. While some protocols recommend extended ligations at low temperatures, we have not found any benefit from overnight ligations at 16 °C when using the ligation conditions described above.

10. If a thermal cycler with adjustable temperature heated lid is available, disable the heated lid during incubations at 25 °C. If heated lid cannot be disabled, leave the lid open for 25 °C incubations.

11. We use a 2.5:1 molar ratio of 5′ to 3′ adapter. If a different concentration of 3′ adapter is used, adjust the amount of 5′ adapter accordingly.

12. The remaining ligated RNA may be stored at −70 °C for future use.

13. Small RNA libraries from biofluids typically require 10–25 total cycles of PCR amplification depending on the type and amount of input RNA. It has been shown that increased amplification does not significantly affect library bias [3, 8]. However, increasing the number of PCR cycles may overamplify the adapter dimer PCR product, causing it to smear in the gel and making it difficult to separate from the desired PCR products. Typically, a single PCR and gel purification step is sufficient to remove most of the adapter dimer from small RNA-containing PCR products. However, for low-input RNA

samples, the adapters are present in such great excess over the input RNA that it can be helpful to perform two consecutive PCR and gel purification steps. The first PCR consists of only a few cycles to prevent overamplifying the excess of adapters. The PCR products are separated by gel electrophoresis and the eluate, enriched for insert-containing PCR products, is then amplified further in a second PCR using universal (not index-specific) PCR primers. A second gel purification is then used to remove residual adapter contaminants.

14. Any high-fidelity PCR master mix can be used for this step. If using a different polymerase, follow the cycling conditions recommended by the manufacturer.

15. Because of the large excess of adapters in low-input small RNA libraries, electrophoretic purification of PCR products is necessary. This can be done using either acrylamide or agarose gels, as long as the gel can sufficiently resolve the insert-containing fragments (~150 bp) from the adapter dimer fragments (126 bp using the adapters specified here). Use of an automated size selection instrument like the PippinPrep, BluePippin, or PippinHT can reduce variability introduced during gel excision.

16. Appropriate size selection parameters will have to be determined by the user based on the method of size selection and the size of the desired inserts. To determine the approximate total size of a library fragment, add the size of the RNA of interest to 126 bp (the size of adapters used in this protocol with no insert).

17. Any high-fidelity PCR master mix can be used for this step. We have found it helpful to perform the second PCR using a qPCR master mix to determine how many cycles to amplify each library. If using a real-time master mix and qPCR machine, use PCR tubes with optical caps.

18. Using the adapters and primers specified in this protocol, a library with predominantly miRNA inserts should have a peak of roughly 150 bp on the Bioanalyzer and adapter dimer contamination will show up as a peak around 126 bp.

19. Oligonucleotides can be ordered from any supplier. Codes shown in Table 1 are as follows: /5rApp/—5′ adenylation; /3ddC/—3′ dideoxycytidine; (N:25252525)(N)(N)(N)—4 hand-mixed degenerate bases, 25% each nucleotide.

20. Oligonucleotide sequences © 2016 Illumina, Inc. All rights reserved. Derivative works created by Illumina customers are authorized for use with Illumina instruments and products only. All other uses are strictly prohibited.

Acknowledgements

This work was supported in part by the NIH Common Fund, Extracellular RNA Communication Consortium (ERCC) 1U01HL126496-01. The authors would like to thank Maria D. Giraldez for helpful suggestions in the preparation of this manuscript.

References

1. Baran-Gale J, Kurtz CL, Erdos MR, Sison C, Young A, Fannin EE, Chines PS, Sethupathy P (2015) Addressing bias in small RNA library preparation for sequencing: a new protocol recovers microRNAs that evade capture by current methods. Front Genet 6:352. https://doi.org/10.3389/fgene.2015.00352

2. Fuchs RT, Sun Z, Zhuang F, Robb GB (2015) Bias in ligation-based small RNA sequencing library construction is determined by adaptor and RNA structure. PLoS One 10(5):e0126049. https://doi.org/10.1371/journal.pone.0126049

3. Jayaprakash AD, Jabado O, Brown BD, Sachidanandam R (2011) Identification and remediation of biases in the activity of RNA ligases in small-RNA deep sequencing. Nucleic Acids Res 39(21):e141. https://doi.org/10.1093/nar/gkr693

4. Zhang Z, Lee JE, Riemondy K, Anderson EM, Yi R (2013) High-efficiency RNA cloning enables accurate quantification of miRNA expression by deep sequencing. Genome Biol 14(10):R109. https://doi.org/10.1186/gb-2013-14-10-r109

5. Sorefan K, Pais H, Hall AE, Kozomara A, Griffiths-Jones S, Moulton V, Dalmay T (2012) Reducing ligation bias of small RNAs in libraries for next generation sequencing. Silence 3(1):4. https://doi.org/10.1186/1758-907X-3-4

6. Viollet S, Fuchs RT, Munafo DB, Zhuang F, Robb GB (2011) T4 RNA ligase 2 truncated active site mutants: improved tools for RNA analysis. BMC Biotechnol 11:72. https://doi.org/10.1186/1472-6750-11-72

7. Song Y, Liu KJ, Wang TH (2014) Elimination of ligation dependent artifacts in T4 RNA ligase to achieve high efficiency and low bias microRNA capture. PLoS One 9(4):e94619. https://doi.org/10.1371/journal.pone.0094619

8. Hafner M, Renwick N, Brown M, Mihailovic A, Holoch D, Lin C, Pena JT, Nusbaum JD, Morozov P, Ludwig J, Ojo T, Luo S, Schroth G, Tuschl T (2011) RNA-ligase-dependent biases in miRNA representation in deep-sequenced small RNA cDNA libraries. RNA 17(9):1697–1712. https://doi.org/10.1261/rna.2799511

Chapter 14

Multiplexed Detection and Quantitation of Extracellular Vesicle RNA Expression Using NanoString

Neha Shukla, Irene K. Yan, and Tushar Patel

Abstract

Several different types of RNA molecules such as microRNAs (miRNAs) have been detected within extracellular vesicles in the circulation. The detection and potential utility of these as disease biomarkers requires the ability to detect their presence with adequate sensitivity and to quantitate their expression. The potential for circulating miRNA to serve as biomarkers can be evaluated through their detection in association with specific disease states. Multiplexed detection of several miRNA simultaneously can be useful for discovery studies. We describe the analysis of miRNA from biological fluids like plasma and serum using the Nanostring nCounter platform. Assays can be used to quantitate the expression of miRNA using direct detection based on hybridization to target specific color-coded probes followed by counting each color-coded barcode digitally.

Key words Extracellular vesicles, Extracellular RNA, miRNA, Biomarkers

1 Introduction

Extracellular RNA hold promise as biomarkers for human diseases, but their evaluation requires the use of sensitive and quantitative methods for the analysis of candidate exRNA. The number of extracellular RNA molecules that can serve as biomarkers is very large, and includes protein coding genes as well as noncoding RNA. The ability to multiplex and perform simultaneous determinations of expression of multiple extracellular RNA is therefore highly desirable for biomarker discovery studies. Multiplexed assays can further support the development of panels that incorporate necessary controls for reproducibility and validation. Additional advantages include the use of lower amounts of input sample and lower material and labor costs.

Herein we provide a protocol for the use of the Nanostring platform for the multiplexed detection and quantitation of extracellular RNA in biological fluids such as serum or plasma. This platform provides a sensitive and reproducible method for the

Tushar Patel (ed.), *Extracellular RNA: Methods and Protocols*, Methods in Molecular Biology, vol. 1740, https://doi.org/10.1007/978-1-4939-7652-2_14, © Springer Science+Business Media, LLC 2018

detection, and quantitation of RNAs that does not require the use of polymerase, reverse transcription or polymerase chain reaction (PCR) amplification [1]. The assays can be adapted for use within a clinical laboratory setting. A limitation of this platform is that the sensitivity of detection may be insufficient to detect low amounts of transcripts. This is of relevance for studies of circulating extracellular RNA biomarkers where the transcripts of interest may be present in very low amounts. Other techniques such as digital PCR may have greater sensitivity, but are less amenable to multiplexing for discovery studies or assay development.

The platform is based on hybridization chemistry and involves the use of capture probes to defined target sites, along with the direct detection of targets by amplification using molecular reporter barcodes. The capture probes are tagged with biotin at the 3'-end, whereas the reporter probes carry a barcode signal at the 5'-end (Fig. 1). These two probes are ~50 bases in size, and hybridize to target RNAs in solution with the formation of a target/probe complex. These complexes are further affinity purified, attached to streptavidin coated slides via biotinylated capture probes, further aligned by voltage and immobilized on the cartridge for imaging. Color-coded barcodes hybridized to samples within the cartridge are counted with a specialized fine microscope and tabulated for each target molecule [2].

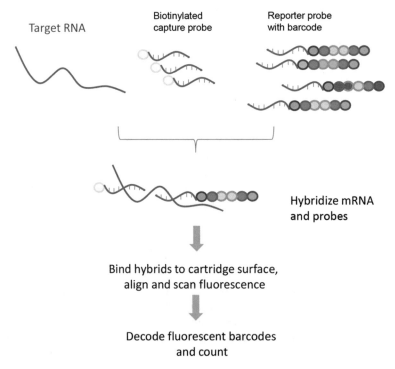

Fig. 1 Overview of Nanostring assay. Two probes for each target gene are used. The hybrids formed between target gene and probes are visualized and decoded based on unique fluorescent barcodes specific for each target gene

The platform can be used for analysis of RNA using customized probe sets that target specific RNAs [3]. Probe sets can include probes for desired housekeeping genes, as well as for other controls such as exogenous RNA, positive or negative controls. Off-the-shelf panels that target groups of preselected RNA are also available. Their use of a premade miRNA expression array which includes probes that target up to 798 miRNA and several controls is described below. These illustrate the capability to perform single-tube multiplexing of extracellular vesicle RNA isolated from plasma for biomarker discovery [4, 5].

2 Materials

2.1 Instruments

1. Bench-top centrifuge.
2. Mini Centrifuge.
3. Mini plate spinner.
4. Thermal cycler.
5. Spectrophotometer.
6. nCounter Prep Station (Nanostring Technologies).
7. nCounter Digital Analyzer (Nanostring Technologies).

2.2 Isolation of Extracellular Vesicle RNA

1. Size exclusion chromatography columns (qEV, iZON science).
2. 1× Phosphate Buffered Saline (PBS).
3. 0.5 M Sodium Hydroxide (NaOH).
4. Total RNA isolation kit (miRCURY-Biofluids, Exiqon).
5. RNA Clean & Concentrator-5 (Zymo).

2.3 RNA Expression Probe Set Array

1. nCounter miRNA Expression Assay Kit (Nanostring Technologies).
2. A customized RNA expression panel could also be used.

2.4 Data Analysis Software

1. nSolver Data Analysis software (Nanostring Technologies).

3 Methods

3.1 Isolation of EV from Plasma Using Size Exclusion Chromatography

1. Centrifuge 1.0 mL plasma sample at 2000 × g for 10 min, transfer to a new tube, and store at −20 °C until use (*see* **Note 1**).
2. Equilibrate the column the first time it is used (*see* **Note 2**). To do so, place the column vertically in a holder and make sure it is leveled. First remove the top-cap carefully, leaving the bottom luer-slip cap in place. Then remove the bottom luer-slip cap, and let the bacteriostatic agent (0.05% sodium azide) flow

through. Rinse the column with 20 mL of PBS added in 2 mL increments to make sure that the column does not run dry. Place the luer-slip cap back and apply additional 2.0 mL of PBS to the top of the column.

3. Sample Application. First remove the top-cap, and with the bottom luer-slip cap on, let 2.0 mL PBS flow through the column. Then add 1.0 mL of the plasma sample, remove the luer-slip cap, and immediately start collecting 500 µL fractions in the microfuge tubes. As the last part of the sample starts to enter the top-filter, begin adding 10 mL of PBS to the top of the column in 2.0 mL intervals. The first six fractions comprise the void volume and do not contain vesicles. The desired vesicle fractions are fractions 7 and 8 (1.0 ml) (*see* **Note 3**).

4. Once vesicle fractions are collected, flush the column with 10 mL of PBS to clean it. Place the luer-slip cap back. Apply an additional 2.0 mL of PBS to the top of the column and store at 4–8 °C.

5. In order to reuse the column, wash it with 10 mL of 0.5 M NaOH, followed by 20 mL PBS (*see* **Note 4**).

3.2 Isolation and Concentration of EV-RNA

1. EV-RNA is isolated from fractions 7 and 8 (*see* **Note 5**).

2. Transfer 1000 µL of supernatant to a new microfuge tube and add 300 µL Lysis solution BF, vortex for 5 s and incubate for 3 min at room temperature.

3. Add 100 µL of Protein Precipitation Solution BF, vortex for 5 s, incubate at room temperature for 1 min, centrifuge at $11,000 \times g$ for 3 min, and then transfer the clear supernatant into a new 5.0 mL collection tube. Add 1350 µL of isopropanol to this sample and vortex for 5 s.

4. Place the mini spin column in a collection tube and load the sample onto it. After incubating at room temperature for 2 min, centrifuge at $11,000 \times g$ for 30 s, and discard the flow through. Place the column back into the collection tube. Keep loading and repeating this step until all of it is used up. Then add 100 µL of Wash Solution 1 BF, centrifuge at $11,000 \times g$ for 30 s, discard the flow through, and replace the column. Repeat this step by adding 700 µL of Wash Solution 2 BF to the column, centrifuge at $11,000 \times g$ for 30 s, discard the flow through, and replace the column. For the final washing step, add 250 µL Wash Solution 2 BF, and centrifuge at $11,000 \times g$ for 2 min.

5. The next step involves elution. Place the column in a new 1.5 mL collection tube and add 50 µL RNase free water directly onto the column membrane, then incubate at room

temperature for 1 min and centrifuge at 11,000 × g for 1 min. For greater extracellular vesicle RNA yield, re-elute the column with 50 µL of RNase free water which gives a total volume of 100 µL of RNA.

6. To concentrate the RNA further, add 200 µL of RNA binding buffer and mix by flicking. Add the same volume of 100% ethanol (300 µL), flick mix, transfer to the Zymo-Spin IC Column with a collection tube, centrifuge at 11,000 × g for 30 s, and discard the flow through. Add 400 µL of RNA Prep Buffer to the column, centrifuge at 11,000 × g for 30 s, and discard the flow through. Wash by adding 700 µL of RNA Wash buffer, then centrifuge at 11,000 × g for 30 s, and discard the flow through again. For the final wash to remove buffer completely, add 400 µL of RNA Wash Buffer, centrifuge at 11,000 × g for 2 min, and discard the flow through. Elute RNA with 8–10 µL of RNase free water directly applied onto the surface of the membrane. For short- and long-term storage, store at −20 and −70 °C, respectively.

3.3 Nanostring Assay for miRNA

1. Sample preparation. Adjust the RNA concentration of the input sample to 33 ng/µL using RNase free water and use 3 µL for the assay (*see* **Note 6**).

2. Prepare controls by adding 1 µL of miRNA Assay Controls to 499 µL of RNase free water (1:500 dilution) in a sterile microfuge tube, vortex briefly, and store on ice.

3. Add 26 µL of nCounter miRNA Tag Reagent and 6.5 µL of the miRNA Assay Controls dilution prepared in **step 2** to 13 µL of Annealing buffer. Mix well by pipetting. Aliquot 3.5 µL of the annealing mastermix into 12 × 0.2 mL strip tubes.

4. Add 3 µL (100 ng) of RNA sample into each tube containing the annealing mastermix mix by flicking and then spin down the solution. Place strip tube in the thermocycler and start the annealing protocol as follows: 94 °C for 1 min, 65 °C for 2 min, 45 °C for 10 min, then hold at 48 °C (*see* **Note 7**).

5. Prepare the ligation master mix by adding 19.5 µL of poly ethylene glycol (PEG) to 13 µL of ligation buffer in a microfuge tube and mix properly by pipetting (*see* **Note 8**).

6. Remove samples from the thermocycler maintaining the thermocycler at 48 °C and then add 2.5 µL of the ligation master mix to each tube, cap the tubes, flick to mix, and spin down.

7. Return the tubes to thermal cycler and incubate at 48 °C for 5 min. Open thermal cycler without removing the tubes, uncap the tubes in the strip, and add 1 µL of ligase to each tube. Mixing with ligase can be skipped.

8. Recap the tubes in the thermocycler immediately and initiate the ligation protocol as follows: 48 °C for 3 min, 47 °C for 3 min, 46 °C for 3 min, 45 °C for 5 min, 65 °C for 10 min, then hold at 4 °C. After the ligation protocol, remove the tubes from the thermocycler, uncap, add 1 μL of Ligation Clean up Enzyme to each tube, flick to mix, and spin down.

9. Return the tubes to the thermocycler and start the purification protocol as follows: 37 °C for 60 min, 70 °C for 10 min, then hold at 4 °C. Remove the tubes from thermocycler and add 40 μL of RNase free water to each tube. Samples can be stored at −20 °C for several weeks before initiating the miRNA CodeSet Hybridization protocol.

10. For the CodeSet Hybridization Assay, prepare thermocycler to 65 °C with the lid set to 70 °C. Prepare a reporter master mix for 12 samples by mixing 130 μL of Reporter CodeSet and 130 μL of hybridization buffer, invert to mix and briefly spin down (*see* **Note 11**). Dispense 20 μL of reporter master mix into each tube of a 12 tube strip. Denature miRNA samples from **step 9** at 85 °C for 5 min on the thermocycler, snap cool for 2 min on ice, and add 5 μL of prepared miRNA sample to reporter mix. Add 5 μL of thawed Capture ProbeSet into each of the 12 strip tubes, cap the tubes, and immediately transfer to 65 °C in the thermocycler. Perform the hybridization assay by incubating at 65 °C for 12–30 h. Maintain samples at 65 °C until **step 6** of the Prep Station.

11. Allow plates and cartridge to come up to room temperature for up to 30 min, prior to starting. Centrifuge reagent plates at $2000 \times g$ for 2 min and look for dark pellets in Row H. Carefully load tips, place reagent plates (remove lids) onto the deck. Replace empty strip tubes into heater slots, insert tip sheaths. Prepare sealed cartridge to room temperature before using and then open cartridge, place on deck, and cautiously insert electrodes making sure not to bend electrodes.

12. Take out samples from the thermocycler, briefly spin down, insert into holder, close heater lid, and immediately initiate protocol. At the end of the protocol, take out the cartridge and immediately seal wells to avoid evaporation using sealing film provided in the kit. Discard sheaths, tips, and plates.

13. Upload customized Reporter Library File (RLF) from the provided USB drive. Upload or create Cartridge Definition File (CDF).

14. Transfer the cartridge to the Digital Analyzer for data collection (*see* **Note 14**). For some older Nanostring instruments, first apply imaging oil to sample cartridge by inserting into the oiler, pressing button, and ensuring that the entire surface is covered. Data collection can take several hours if the reporter

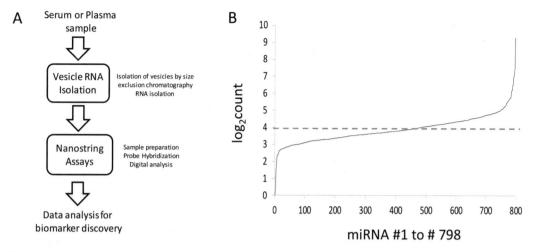

Fig. 2 (**a**) Scheme for circulating EV RNA biomarker discovery using multiplexed Nanostring detection. (**b**) Expression levels of 798 miRNA from circulating EV RNA in a patient with hepatocellular cancer. The *dotted line* depicts background limit and represents two times the upper limit of detected counts in negative controls

counts are higher. Once run is completed, download and transfer data in the form of Reporter Code Count (RCC) files using provided USB drive (*see* **Note 15**, Fig. 2).

3.4 Data Analysis

1. The RCC files can be analyzed using the nSolver software. In order to analyze expression data, normalization to expression of controls or housekeeping genes will be necessary.

2. Background correction can be performed based on cutoff derived from counts detected on negative controls, for example by subtracting the mean ± 2 standard deviations of the mean of negative controls, or by using the upper limit of counts detected in any negative control as a cutoff. Background subtraction may improve fold-change estimation.

3. Normalization could be performed using the geometric mean of positive controls. Code set content normalization with the geometric mean for all genes is recommended.

4 Notes

1. When working with plasma or serum samples, avoid the use of hemolyzed samples because traces of red blood cells can affect RNA expression profile. Obtain cell-free starting material by centrifugation at $300 \times g$ for 10 min.

2. The size exclusion chromatography column works best at 4–8 °C and can also be used to isolate extracellular vesicle fractions from various biological fluids like serum, plasma, saliva, urine, and cell culture media.

3. During sample application to chromatography columns, waiting until the last of the sample enters the top-filter avoids sample dilution.

4. Cleaning the column with 10 mL of 0.5 M NaOH helps in removal of precipitated proteins, nonspecifically bound proteins, and lipoproteins. 20 mL of a nonionic detergent solution like 0.1% Triton X-100 followed by 20–30 mL of PBS can also be considered for removal of strongly bound proteins, lipoproteins, and lipids.

5. Vesicle fractions can be analyzed using nanoparticle tracking analysis. The protein concentration can be determined using BCA Assay and RNA concentration can be estimated spectrophotometrically. The vesicle elution should peak at fractions 7 + 8. This may need to be verified for different conditions.

6. The quality of the input RNA used for the assay is of paramount importance and can be assessed spectrophotometrically. An absorbance 260 nm/280 nm ratio of ≥ 1.9 and 260 nm/230 nm ratio of ≥ 1.8 is recommended. Residual assay reagents like lysis buffer, phenol, wash buffer, or ethanol are potential contaminants which can alter assay performance by inhibiting the enzymatic reactions and purification.

7. Maintaining temperature of thermocycler is critical.

8. PEG should be pipetted very slowly to ensure accurate measurement because of its viscosity.

9. For efficient dispensing and keeping track of master mix, ligase, or any other critical solvents, it is helpful to line up 12 tips in front, discarding each tip after use.

10. Avoid samples at room temperature to reduce background counts.

11. For efficient hybridization, thaw Reporter and capture probe sets appropriately so that no precipitates are present. Heat at 75 °C for 10 min, and cool at room temperature before use.

12. Mix by flicking and inverting tubes, avoid harsh pipetting and vortexing during the assay to prevent shearing the probes.

13. If the Prep Station has not been in use for more than 3 weeks, a calibration run is recommended before performing the assay.

14. Cartridge can be stored for up to 7 days at 4 °C before reading.

15. When inserting cartridge into Digital Analyzer, it should be ensured that it is pressed down flat, to the feet of the cartridge carrier.

16. Once the RLF file is uploaded from the provided USB drive, it remains on the Digital Analyzer for use in subsequent runs.

17. Normalization of extracellular vesicle miRNA expression using endogenous and exogenous controls is necessary but confounded by low expression in serum samples, and by considerable variation in plasma samples.

18. For detailed additional discussion of statistical issues, refer to Refs. [6–8].

Acknowledgments

This work was supported by the Office of the Director, National Institutes of Health (USA) through award UH3 TR000884. We acknowledge the expert assistance of Caitlyn Foerst and thank the members of our laboratories for their contributions.

Disclosures: None.

References

1. Tsang HF, Xue VW, Koh SP, Chiu YM, Ng LP, Wong SC (2017) NanoString, a novel digital color-coded barcode technology: current and future applications in molecular diagnostics. Expert Rev Mol Diagn 17(1):95–103. https://doi.org/10.1080/14737159.2017.1268533

2. Geiss GK, Bumgarner RE, Birditt B, Dahl T, Dowidar N, Dunaway DL, Fell HP, Ferree S, George RD, Grogan T, James JJ, Maysuria M, Mitton JD, Oliveri P, Osborn JL, Peng T, Ratcliffe AL, Webster PJ, Davidson EH, Hood L, Dimitrov K (2008) Direct multiplexed measurement of gene expression with color-coded probe pairs. Nat Biotechnol 26(3):317–325. https://doi.org/10.1038/nbt1385

3. Markowitz J, Abrams Z, Jacob NK, Zhang X, Hassani JN, Latchana N, Wei L, Regan KE, Brooks TR, Uppati SR, Levine KM, Bekaii-Saab T, Kendra KL, Lesinski GB, Howard JH, Olencki T, Payne PR, Carson WE 3rd (2016) MicroRNA profiling of patient plasma for clinical trials using bioinformatics and biostatistical approaches. Onco Targets Ther 9:5931–5941. https://doi.org/10.2147/OTT.S106288

4. Das K, Chan XB, Epstein D, Teh BT, Kim KM, Kim ST, Park SH, Kang WK, Rozen S, Lee J, Tan P (2016) NanoString expression profiling identifies candidate biomarkers of RAD001 response in metastatic gastric cancer. ESMO Open 1(1):e000009. https://doi.org/10.1136/esmoopen-2015-000009

5. Oikonomopoulos A, Polytarchou C, Joshi S, Hommes DW, Iliopoulos D (2016) Identification of circulating MicroRNA signatures in Crohn's disease using the Nanostring nCounter technology. Inflamm Bowel Dis 22(9):2063–2069. https://doi.org/10.1097/MIB.0000000000000883

6. Wang H, Horbinski C, Wu H, Liu Y, Sheng S, Liu J, Weiss H, Stromberg AJ, Wang C (2016) NanoStringDiff: a novel statistical method for differential expression analysis based on NanoString nCounter data. Nucleic Acids Res 44(20):e151. https://doi.org/10.1093/nar/gkw677

7. Veldman-Jones MH, Brant R, Rooney C, Geh C, Emery H, Harbron CG, Wappett M, Sharpe A, Dymond M, Barrett JC, Harrington EA, Marshall G (2015) Evaluating robustness and sensitivity of the NanoString technologies nCounter platform to enable multiplexed gene expression analysis of clinical samples. Cancer Res 75(13):2587–2593. https://doi.org/10.1158/0008-5472.CAN-15-0262

8. Jung SH, Sohn I (2014) Statistical issues in the design and analysis of nCounter projects. Cancer Inform 13(Suppl 7):35–43. https://doi.org/10.4137/CIN.S16343

Chapter 15

Milk-derived Extracellular Vesicles for Therapeutic Delivery of Small Interfering RNAs

Akiko Matsuda and Tushar Patel

Abstract

As endogenous biological nanoparticles capable of uptake by cells, extracellular vesicles (EVs) have the capacity to deliver their RNA cargo to recipient cells. The use of EVs as a drug delivery system remains in its infancy, and there are several barriers to the use of EV for this purpose. Amongst these is the need to ensure that adequate amounts of EV are available. The use of milk-derived EV provides a scalable approach and loading of these EVs with RNA is possible with the use of chemical transfection reagents. This method describes the use of milk-derived EV for delivery of small interfering RNA. These EVs were shown to be taken up by hepatocellular carcinoma cells in vitro, with a reduction in the expression of target gene.

Key words Drug delivery, Extracellular vesicles, Milk, siRNA, Drug loading method, Lipofection, Ultracentrifugation

1 Introduction

Extracellular vesicles (EVs) are nano-sized membrane vesicles released by many different types of cells. There are several different types of EVs, such as exosomes, microvesicles (MVs), or apoptotic bodies (ABs) that vary in their intracellular origin and size [1–3]. The cargo of EVs comprises coding and noncoding RNAs (e.g., mRNA, microRNA, and long noncoding RNA), lipids, and proteins [4, 5]. EVs can contribute to intercellular communication through their uptake by recipient cells and by transferring their cargo between cells which can result in modulation of gene or protein expression [1, 6, 7]. Their ability for uptake and their physiological contribution to intercellular communication has generated interest in the use of EVs as natural drug delivery vehicles that could be loaded with desired therapeutic molecules.

EVs have many features of an ideal drug delivery vehicle. They are widely distributed in biological fluids such as blood [8], urine [9], and breast milk [10], and thus are well tolerated in a variety of environments. Importantly, EVs have been shown to cross natural

Tushar Patel (ed.), *Extracellular RNA: Methods and Protocols*, Methods in Molecular Biology, vol. 1740,
https://doi.org/10.1007/978-1-4939-7652-2_15, © Springer Science+Business Media, LLC 2018

barriers, such as the plasma membrane and the blood–brain barrier, to deliver their cargo into recipient cells [1, 11, 12]. In addition, the membrane of EVs could be modified to enhance cell type-specific targeting. In an early report of the use of EVs to deliver exogenous siRNA, dendritic cells were transfected with targeting peptide expressing plasmids. These cells produced EVs with the targeting peptide that could be efficiently taken up by recipient cells [13]. Immunogenicity of synthetic nucleic acid or delivery vehicles such as liposome are a barrier for drug delivery. However, EVs may have reduced immunogenic potential particularly when autologous EVs are used. Several clinical trials using EVs for immunotherapy have demonstrated the safety of EV administration in humans [14–16].

EVs can be isolated from several different types of body fluids such as serum, ascites, saliva, or milk [17]. Herein we have described the isolation of EV from bovine milk. There are several advantages for the use of milk-derived EV as a drug delivery carrier such as scalability, and cost-effectiveness. In toxicology studies, the use of milk-derived EV has been well tolerated and we did not observe any genotoxic effects in vitro [18]. The presence of a lipid bilayer membrane makes loading of exogenous cargo into EVs challenging, but several methods have been described. One approach is based on donor cell transfection with nucleic acid constructs that can be transferred or translated into products that are loaded onto EV released by these cells [19–21]. Another approach involves loading of EVs after their isolation using methods such as electroporation [13, 22–25], incubation [26, 27], or the use of chemical transfection reagents [22, 23]. A potential consideration for the use of electroporation to load nucleic acids is that, under certain conditions, siRNA aggregates formed during the electroporation process may falsely be interpreted as siRNA loaded into EVs [28]. Moreover, EV integrity and nucleic acid structure may be affected by the electroporation [29]. Chemical-based transfection reagents have also been used to load EV with siRNA [22, 23].

In this method, we provide a method for isolation of EV from bovine milk and loading with siRNA using chemical-based transfection. The efficiency of chemical-based transfection may be affected if leftover micelles (with captured siRNA) are present within the resulting EV preparations [30]. Toxicity is a challenge with the use of chemical reagents such as lipofectamine, and cationic micelles that have a high positive surface charge. Compared with nonionic micelles, cationic micelles can decrease cell viability and increase release of pro-inflammatory cytokines [31]. In this method, leftover Lipofectamine-siRNA complex are removed from EV loaded with siRNA by ultracentrifugation. Consistent with this, the zeta potential of EVs loaded with siRNA was similar to that of source EVs. The efficacy of use of milk EV for siRNA delivery was confirmed in vitro by observing that B-catenin expression was decreased in HepG2 cells incubated with EVs loaded with B-catenin siRNA compared with control EVs loaded with scr-siRNA after 48 h.

2   Materials

2.1   EV isolation and Characterization

1. Fat free bovine milk.
2. Phosphate buffered saline (PBS).
3. Ca^{2+} free EDTA.
4. 3.0 M HCL.
5. 3.0 M NaOH.
6. Polycarbonate ultracentrifuge tubes (25 × 89 mm, Beckman Coulter).
7. 0.22 and 0.45 μm PES vacuum filters.
8. Beckman Coulter Optima™ L-80XP Ultracentrifuge.
9. Type 70Ti Rotor.
10. pH Meter.
11. NanoSight LM10 (NanoSight, Amesbury, UK) for particle size and quantitation.
12. Transmission Electron Microscope (optional, for validation).

2.2   Loading of siRNA to EV

1. β-Catenin siRNA (Qiagen, Hs_CTNNB1_3) (*see* **Note1**).
2. Lipofectamine 2000 (Invitrogen).
3. Opti-MEM.
4. Phosphate buffered saline (PBS) 200 ml.
5. Ultra-Clear Centrifuge Tubes (11 × 60 mm, Beckman Coulter).
6. Beckman Coulter Optima™ L-80XP Ultracentrifuge.
7. Type SW 60Ti Rotor.
8. Zeta potential analyzer (Litesizer™ 500, Anton Paar) (optional).

2.3   Labeling of EV and siRNA

1. β-Catenin siRNA (Qiagen, Hs_CTNNB1_3).
2. PKH67 Fluorescent Cell Linker Kit (Sigma-Aldrich).
3. Pierce RNA 3′ end biotinylation Kit (ThermoFisher Scientific).
4. 1% bovine serum albumin (BSA).
5. Ultra-Clear Centrifuge Tubes (14 × 89 mm, Beckman Coulter).
6. Beckman Coulter Optima™ L-80XP Ultracentrifuge.
7. Type SW 41Ti Rotor.

2.4 Observation of Cellular Uptake of EV Loaded with siRNA

1. Milk-derived EVs labeled with PKH67.
2. Biotinylated B-catenin siRNA.
3. HepG2 cells.
4. Dulbecco's modified Eagle's medium (DMEM) supplemented with 10% fetal bovine serum (FBS).
5. Biotin Primary antibody.
6. Alexa Fluor 488-Streptavidin (Invitrogen).
7. Prolong Gold antifade reagent containing nuclear stain DAPI (Life Technologies).
8. 4% paraformaldehyde.
9. Lab-Tek chamber slide, 4 wells (collagen coated).
10. Confocal microscope (Carl Zeiss LSM510).

2.5 Immunoblot Analysis of Target Expression in Recipient Cells

1. Milk-derived EVs (5×10^{12} particles/ml).
2. β-Catenin siRNA (Qiagen, Hs_CTNNB1_3).
3. HepG2 cells.
4. Dulbecco's modified Eagle's medium (DMEM) supplemented with 10% fetal bovine serum (FBS).
5. 6 well plate (Falcon).
6. cOmplete™ Lysis-M EDTA-free (Sigma-Aldrich).
7. BCA Protein Assays (ThermoFisher Scientific).
8. NuPAGE® Novex® Bis-Tris Mini Gels (ThermoFisher Scien-tific).
9. NuPAGE™ MES SDS Running Buffer (ThermoFisher Scien-tific).
10. iBlot™ 2 Transfer Stacks, PVDF, mini (ThermoFisher Scien-tific).
11. Odyssey Blocking Buffer (LI-COR Biosciences).
12. PBS-Tween 20 (PBST, 1 L PBS supplemented with 2 ml Tween20, Sigma-Aldrich).
13. β-Catenin primary antibody (E-5, sc-7963, Santa Cruz Bio-technology, Inc.).
14. Mouse Secondary antibody.
15. FLUOstar Omega (BMG Labtech).
16. LI-COR Odyssey infrared fluorescent imaging system (LI-COR).

3 Methods

3.1 EV Isolation and Characterization

1. Dilute the milk with an equal amount of PBS (For large scale could use 200 ml milk + 200 ml PBS).

2. Centrifuge at $12,000 \times g$ for 30 min at 4 °C.

3. Carefully remove the top layer using a pipet-aid and transfer the supernatant to a new beaker. Do not disturb the pellet (*see* **Note 2**).

4. Treat supernatant with Ca^{2+} free EDTA, mixing gently using a stir bar, until the solution becomes yellow and nearly clear (*see* **Note 3**).

5. Adjust the pH of the solution to 4.2 with 3.0 M HCL and allow the solution to precipitate for 10–30 min at 4 °C.

6. Centrifuge the supernatant at $10,000 \times g$ for 30 min at 4 °C.

7. Transfer the supernatant to a clean beaker without disturbing the pellet.

8. Filter the supernatant with a 0.45 µm PES vacuum filter.

9. Adjust the pH of the solution to 7.0 using 3.0 M NaOH.

10. Filter the supernatant using a 0.22 µm PES vacuum filter. Store the supernatant at 4 °C for up to 2 days.

11. Transfer to ultracentrifuge tubes and spin at $100,000 \times g$ for 70 min at 4 °C (*see* **Note 4**).

12. Discard the supernatant completely and wash with PBS. Spin at $100,000 \times g$ for 70 min at 4 °C.

13. Discard the supernatant and aspirate all remaining PBS. Resuspend the pellet in 250–500 µl PBS (*see* **Note 5**).

14. (Optional validation) Transmission electron microscopy could be performed to examine the morphology and size of the isolated EV (*see* Fig. 1).

15. Measure the number of particles and the particle sizes using Nanoparticle Tracking Analysis (Nanosight) and adjust concentrations as needed for the next steps (*see* Fig. 2 and **Note 6**).

3.2 Loading of siRNA into EV

1. In a 1.5 ml microcentrifuge tube, prepare 0.5 µM of β-catenin siRNA in 25 µl Opti-MEM and vortex lightly to mix (*see* **Note 7**).

2. In another 1.5 ml microcentrifuge tube, prepare 2.0 µl Lipofectamine 2000 in 25 µl Opti-MEM and vortex lightly to mix.

3. Mix an equal volume of plasmid and Lipofectamine solution, and incubate for 10 min at room temperature.

4. Add mixture to 50 µl EV (5×10^{12} particles/ml) in an ultracentrifuge tube (11×60 mm), pipette gently, and incubate 30 min at room temperature (*see* **Note 8**).

5. After incubation, dilute the samples with 4 ml PBS.

6. Ultracentrifuge at $100,000 \times g$ for 70 min at 4 °C using an SW 60Ti rotor (*see* **Note 9**).

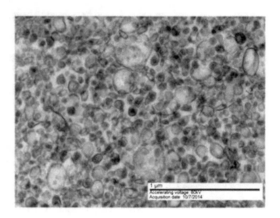

Fig. 1 Transmission electron microscopic image of milk-derived EV. Most of the EVs were in the size range of 100–200 nm

a

b

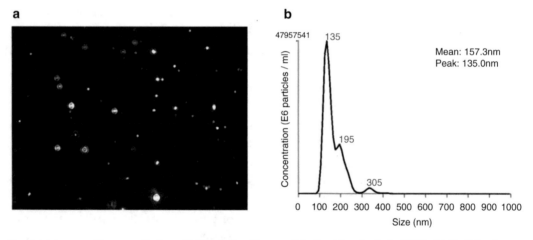

Fig. 2 (**a**) Image of laser scattering of MNV during Nanoparticle Tracking Analysis (NTA). (**b**) Particle size per concentration quantitated using NTA. Milk-derived EV with a mean size of 157.3 nm and a peak size of 135.0 nm

7. Remove the supernatant and resuspend the pellet in 50 μl PBS (*see* **Note 10**).

8. (Optional validation) Measure zeta potential of EV, EV loaded with siRNA or Lipofectamine using a zeta potential analyzer (the Litesizer™ 500, Anton Paar) to evaluate whether siRNA-Lipofectamine complexes are removed by ultracentrifugation (*see* Fig. **3**).

3.3 Labeling of EV and siRNA

1. Add 50 μl EV (5×10^{12} particles/ml) in PBS up to 2000 μl of Diluent C and mix gently in a centrifuge tube (14 × 89 mm) (*see* **Note 11**).

2. Prepare 2 ml of 2× dye working solution by adding 8 μl of PKH67 dye to 1992 μl of Diluent C and mix.

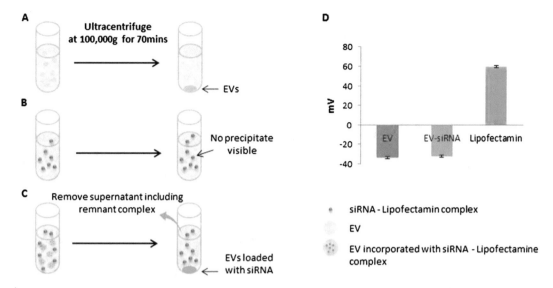

Fig. 3 (**a–c**) Schematic overview of studies. (**a**) EVs, (**b**) siRNA-Lipofectamine complex, or (**c**) EVs loaded with siRNA were subject to ultracentrifugation. Subsequently, a pellet was present with EV or with EV loaded with siRNA (**a**, **c**), but not with siRNA-Lipofectamine complexes. (**d**) Zeta potential of EV, EV loaded with siRNA or Lipofectamine was measured using a zeta potential analyzer (the Litesizer™ 500, Anton Paar). A high positive charge was observed with Lipofectamine (59.58 ± 0.95 mV), whereas EV or EV loaded with siRNA had a negative zeta potential (−33.64 ± 0.83 and −32.28 ± 1.25 mV, respectively)

3. Add 2 ml of 2× dye to EV with 2 ml of Diluent C and mix gently.

4. Incubate at room temperature with periodic mixing for 15 min.

5. Stop the staining by adding 4 ml of 1% BSA and incubate for 1 min at room temperature.

6. After incubation, dilute the samples with 4 ml PBS.

7. Ultracentrifuge at $100,000 \times g$ for 70 min at 4 °C.

8. Remove supernatant, and resuspend the pellet with 50 μl PBS.

9. Prepare biotinylated β-catenin siRNA using the Pierce RNA 3′ end biotinylation Kit and following the instructions provided by the manufacturers (ThermoFisher Scientific).

3.4 Observation of Cellular Uptake EV Loaded with siRNA

1. Culture HepG2 cells (3×10^4 cells/well) on collagen coated 4 chamber slides in DMEM with 10% FBS for 24 h.

2. Prepare 50 μl PKH labeled EV loaded with β-catenin siRNA (5×10^{12} particles/ml) using the procedure described above in Subheadings 3.2 and 3.3.

3. For negative controls, prepare 50 μl PKH labeled EV (5×10^{12} particles/ml) without siRNA and 0.5 μM biotinylated β-catenin siRNA in 50 μl Opti-MEM.

4. Prepare 50 μl biotinylated β-catenin siRNA and Lipofectamine complex solution for positive control according to the procedure described in **steps 1** and **2** in Subheading 3.2.

5. Add 25 μl of sample to each well of HepG2 cells and incubate for 24 h.

6. After incubation, wash cells briefly with PBS.

7. Aspirate PBS, and incubate cells with 4% paraformaldehyde for 15 min at room temperature.

8. Aspirate fixative, and rinse three times with FBS, 5 min each.

9. Block cells with blocking buffer for 1 h at room temperature.

10. Incubate cells overnight with Biotin Primary Antibody (1:400).

11. Incubate cells with Alexa Fluor 488-Streptavidin (1:400) for 30 min at room temperature.

12. Wash 3× with PBS, 5 min each.

13. Coverslip slides with Prolong Gold Antifade Reagent with DAPI.

14. Image cells using a Confocal Microscope.

3.5 Immunoblot Analysis of Target Expression in Recipient Cells

1. Culture HepG2 cells (3×10^5 cells/well) on a collagen coated 6-well plate in DMEM with 10% FBS for 24 h.

2. Prepare EV loaded with siRNA sample at four different B-catenin siRNA concentrations (12.5, 25.0, 50.0, and 100 nM) according to the procedures described above.

3. For a negative control, prepare an unmodified EV sample (mixture of 50 μl EVs and 50 μl Opti-MEM, and perform ultracentrifugation as noted in **step 6** in Subheading 3.2).

4. For positive control, prepare the siRNA-Lipofectamine complex as in **step 3** in Subheading 3.2.

5. Add 50 μl sample to each well (2 ml culture media) and incubate for 48 h.

6. Wash cells with cold PBS twice and add 250 μl cell lysate buffer to each well.

7. Scrape cells with comb and collect cell lysate in a microcentrifuge tube.

8. Measure protein concentration using BCA protein assay kit according to the kit instructions.

9. Incubate 20 μg protein with loading buffer in each sample for 10 min at 70 °C.

10. Load each protein sample on the gel and run for 35 min at 200 V.

11. Transfer protein on the gel to membrane for 10 min by electroblotting method.

12. Incubate membrane in 10 ml blocking buffer for 30 min with shaking.

13. Incubate membrane with β-catenin primary antibody diluted with 5 ml blocking buffer (1:1000) at 4 °C overnight with shaking.

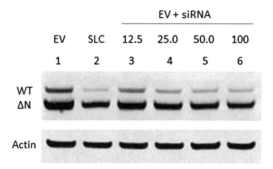

Fig. 4 Immunoblot assay for β-catenin protein, wild type (WT) and ΔN truncated mutant (ΔN). HepG2 cells were incubated with EV (*lane 1*), β-catenin siRNA-lipofectamine complexes (SLC) (*lane 2*), EV loaded with β-catenin siRNA (12.5, 25.0, 50.0, and 100 nM, respectively in *lanes 3, 4, 5,* and *6*). After transfer of siRNA via EV, β-catenin expression was decreased in a dose dependent manner (*lane 3–6*) compared with negative controls (*lane 1*). 5.0×10^{11} particles were loaded in each of the EV containing wells

14. Wash membrane with PBST three times and incubate for 10 min in RT with shaking.

15. After washing with PBST again, incubate with secondary antibody (1:10,000) for 30 min at RT with shaking.

16. After washing three times with PBST, scan the membrane using Odyssey infrared system and quantify the fluorescence (*see* Fig. 4).

4   Notes

1. This method describes the use of validated and optimized siRNA to β-catenin. For use with other siRNA, efficacy and concentration would need to be established to ensure that adequate suppression of target gene expression occurs.

2. Removal of supernatant from the top using a pipet-aid will provide a purer sample than decanting by avoiding admixing with pelleted material.

3. A total of 13–15 ml Ca^{2+} free EDTA may be needed for this step.

4. When supernatant is transferred to a tube, the tube weights should be balanced prior to ultracentrifugation.

5. A recommended dilution volume of PBS is 250–500 μl. The appropriate EV concentration will be based on needs for the next step. Please note that the EV pellet may remain as a precipitate if the volume used is too low.

6. In place of measuring particle number, protein concentration could be assessed as a measure of the amount of EV present, and used for the calculations in subsequent steps.

7. The concentration of the lipofectamine will need to be modified if a higher or different concentration of siRNA is used.

8. The efficacy of siRNA delivery may be reduced if the EV count is low. For in vitro validation, we evaluated target gene expression after siRNA transfer via EV by immunoblotting and observed a decrease in expression.

9. Other rotors may be appropriate based on the total reaction volume.

10. After ultracentrifugation, the recovery of EVs will be reduced by 20–30%. We recommend repeat measurement of EV particle number after ultracentrifugation.

11. In order to check for carryover of dye, a control solution with PBS in Diluent is recommended.

Acknowledgements

This work was supported by the National Institutes of Health (USA) Office of the Director through grant UH3 TR000884. We acknowledge the expert assistance of Caitlyn Foerst and thank the members of our laboratories for their contributions.

References

1. Valadi H, Ekstrom K, Bossios A, Sjostrand M, Lee JJ, Lotvall JO (2007) Exosome-mediated transfer of mRNAs and microRNAs is a novel mechanism of genetic exchange between cells. Nat Cell Biol 9:654–659

2. Skog J, Wurdinger T, van Rijn S, Meijer DH, Gainche L, Sena-Esteves M et al (2008) Glioblastoma microvesicles transport RNA and proteins that promote tumour growth and provide diagnostic biomarkers. Nat Cell Biol 10:1470–1476

3. Duijvesz D, Luider T, Bangma CH, Jenster G (2011) Exosomes as biomarker treasure chests for prostate cancer. Eur Urol 59:823–831

4. Raposo G, Stoorvogel W (2013) Extracellular vesicles: exosomes, microvesicles, and friends. J Cell Biol 200:373–383

5. van Dommelen SM, Vader P, Lakhal S, Kooijmans SA, van Solinge WW, Wood MJ et al (2012) Microvesicles and exosomes: opportunities for cell-derived membrane vesicles in drug delivery. J Control Release 161: 635–644

6. Ratajczak J, Miekus K, Kucia M, Zhang J, Reca R, Dvorak P et al (2006) Embryonic stem cell-derived microvesicles reprogram hematopoietic progenitors: evidence for horizontal transfer of mRNA and protein delivery. Leukemia 20: 847–856

7. Pegtel DM, Cosmopoulos K, Thorley-Lawson DA, van Eijndhoven MA, Hopmans ES, Lindenberg JL et al (2010) Functional delivery of viral miRNAs via exosomes. Proc Natl Acad Sci U S A 107:6328–6333

8. MP C (2005) Exosomal-like vesicles are present in human blood plasma. Int Immunol 17: 879–887

9. Zhou H, Pisitkun T, Aponte A, Yuen PS, Hoffert JD, Yasuda H et al (2006) Exosomal Fetuin-A identified by proteomics: a novel urinary biomarker for detecting acute kidney injury. Kidney Int 70:1847–1857

10. Admyre C, Johansson SM, Qazi KR, Filen JJ, Lahesmaa R, Norman M et al (2007) Exosomes with immune modulatory features are present in human breast milk. J Immunol 179:1969–1978

11. Andre F, Chaput N, Schartz NE, Flament C, Aubert N, Bernard J et al (2004) Exosomes as potent cell-free peptide-based vaccine. I. Dendritic cell-derived exosomes transfer functional MHC class I/peptide complexes to dendritic cells. J Immunol 172:2126–2136

12. Thery C, Duban L, Segura E, Veron P, Lantz O, Amigorena S (2002) Indirect activation of naive CD4+ T cells by dendritic cell-derived exosomes. Nat Immunol 3:1156–1162

13. Alvarez-Erviti L, Seow Y, Yin H, Betts C, Lakhal S, Wood MJ (2011) Delivery of siRNA to the mouse brain by systemic injection of targeted exosomes. Nat Biotechnol 29:341–345

14. Escudier B, Dorval T, Chaput N, Andre F, Caby MP, Novault S et al (2005) Vaccination of metastatic melanoma patients with autologous dendritic cell (DC) derived-exosomes: results of thefirst phase I clinical trial. J Transl Med 3:10

15. Morse MA, Garst J, Osada T, Khan S, Hobeika A, Clay TM et al (2005) A phase I study of dexosome immunotherapy in patients with advanced non-small cell lung cancer. J Transl Med 3:9

16. Dai S, Wei D, Wu Z, Zhou X, Wei X, Huang H et al (2008) Phase I clinical trial of autologous ascites-derived exosomes combined with GM-CSF for colorectal cancer. Mol Ther 16:782–790

17. Munagala R, Aqil F, Jeyabalan J, Gupta RC (2016) Bovine milk-derived exosomes for drug delivery. Cancer Lett 371:48–61

18. Maji S, Yan IK, Parasramka M, Mohankumar S, Matsuda A, Patel T (2017) In vitro toxicology studies of extracellular vesicles. J Appl Toxicol 37:310–318

19. Kosaka N, Iguchi H, Yoshioka Y, Takeshita F, Matsuki Y, Ochiya T (2010) Secretory mechanisms and intercellular transfer of microRNAs in living cells. J Biol Chem 285:17442–17452

20. Kosaka N, Iguchi H, Yoshioka Y, Hagiwara K, Takeshita F, Ochiya T (2012) Competitive interactions of cancer cells and normal cells via secretory microRNAs. J Biol Chem 287:1397–1405

21. Pan Q, Ramakrishnaiah V, Henry S, Fouraschen S, de Ruiter PE, Kwekkeboom J et al (2012) Hepatic cell-to-cell transmission of small silencing RNA can extend the therapeutic reach of RNA interference (RNAi). Gut 61:1330–1339

22. Wahlgren J, De LKT, Brisslert M, Vaziri Sani F, Telemo E, Sunnerhagen P et al (2012) Plasma exosomes can deliver exogenous short interfering RNA to monocytes and lymphocytes. Nucleic Acids Res 40:e130

23. Shtam TA, Kovalev RA, Varfolomeeva EY, Makarov EM, Kil YV, Filatov MV (2013) Exosomes are natural carriers of exogenous siRNA to human cells in vitro. Cell Commun Signal 11:88

24. Hood JL, Scott MJ, Wickline SA (2014) Maximizing exosome colloidal stability following electroporation. Anal Biochem 448:41–49

25. Tian Y, Li S, Song J, Ji T, Zhu M, Anderson GJ et al (2014) A doxorubicin delivery platform using engineered natural membrane vesicle exosomes for targeted tumor therapy. Biomaterials 35:2383–2390

26. Sun D, Zhuang X, Xiang X, Liu Y, Zhang S, Liu C et al (2010) A novel nanoparticle drug delivery system: the anti-inflammatory activity of curcumin is enhanced when encapsulated in exosomes. Mol Ther 18:1606–1614

27. Jang SC, Kim OY, Yoon CM, Choi DS, Roh TY, Park J et al (2013) Bioinspired exosome-mimetic nanovesicles for targeted delivery of chemotherapeutics to malignant tumors. ACS Nano 7:7698–7710

28. Kooijmans SA, Stremersch S, Braeckmans K, de Smedt SC, Hendrix A, Wood MJ et al (2013) Electroporation-induced siRNA precipitation obscures the efficiency of siRNA loading into extracellular vesicles. J Control Release 172:229–238

29. Jiang L, Vader P, Schiffelers RM (2017) Extracellular vesicles for nucleic acid delivery: progress and prospects for safe RNA-based gene therapy. Gene Ther 24:157–166

30. Johnsen KB, Gudbergsson JM, Skov MN, Pilgaard L, Moos T, Duroux M (2014) A comprehensive overview of exosomes as drug delivery vehicles – endogenous nanocarriers for targeted cancer therapy. Biochim Biophys Acta 1846:75–87

31. Elsabahy M, Zhang S, Zhang F, Deng ZJ, Lim YH, Wang H et al (2013) Surface charges and shell crosslinks each play significant roles in mediating degradation, biofouling, cytotoxicity and immunotoxicity for polyphosphoester-based nanoparticles. Sci Rep 3:3313

Chapter 16

Loading of Extracellular Vesicles with Hydrophobically Modified siRNAs

Marie-Cecile Didiot, Reka A. Haraszti, Neil Aronin, and Anastasia Khvorova

Abstract

Delivery represents a significant barrier to the clinical advancement of oligonucleotide therapeutics. Small, endogenous extracellular vesicles (EVs) have the potential to act as oligonucleotide delivery vehicles, but robust and scalable methods for loading RNA therapeutic cargo into vesicles are lacking. Here we describe the efficient loading of hydrophobically modified siRNAs (hsiRNAs) into EVs upon co-incubation, without altering vesicle size distribution or integrity. This method is expected to advance the development of EV-based therapies for the treatment of a broad range of disorders.

Key words Extracellular vesicles, Oligonucleotide therapeutics, Hydrophobically modified siRNA, RNA interference

1 Introduction

Oligonucleotide therapeutics (ONTs) represent a new class of drug targeting RNA or DNA, thus preventing expression of the protein responsible for the disease phenotype. The recent progress in the chemistry of therapeutic oligonucleotides enables design of fully metabolically stabilized siRNAs, which maintain an ability to efficiently enter into the RISC complex [1]. Hydrophobically modified siRNAs (hsiRNAs) are asymmetric oligonucleotides with chemical modifications that improve stability and promote cellular internalization [2] . A cholesterol moiety, conjugated to the 3′ end of the passenger strand, enables rapid membrane association, and the single-stranded phosphorothioate tail promotes cellular internalization by a mechanism similar to that used by conventional antisense oligonucleotides [3]. We have recently demonstrated that these compounds efficiently bind cellular membranes, enter cells, and induce potent gene silencing [2, 4, 5]. Upon local injection, their spread is low and efficacy is mostly limited to tissues immediately surrounding the site of administration [4].

Tushar Patel (ed.), *Extracellular RNA: Methods and Protocols*, Methods in Molecular Biology, vol. 1740,
https://doi.org/10.1007/978-1-4939-7652-2_16, © Springer Science+Business Media, LLC 2018

Endogenously produced extracellular vesicles (EVs) mediate intercellular communication by transferring lipids, proteins, and functional RNAs between cells and play a crucial role in physiological and pathological processes [6, 7]. Thus, EVs have recently raised considerable interest to serve as a novel vehicle for therapeutic oligonucleotides delivery [8]. Methods of loading oligonucleotides into exosomes have included electroporation [9, 10] or overexpression of siRNA in exosome-producing cells [11–13]. Though both methods have been shown to promote cellular uptake and target gene silencing, neither can be easily controlled or scaled for production [14]. Moreover, electroporation was shown to disrupt exosome integrity [14], thereby dampening enthusiasm for the potential utility of exosomes for therapeutic oligonucleotide delivery.

Here, we describe a method exploring the membrane binding ability of hydrophobically modified siRNA to promote loading of EVs with the hsiRNAs. Following EVs purification from cell culture conditioned medium, simple co-incubation of hsiRNAs with EVs is an efficient method for their productive and controlled loading of EVs. We have demonstrated the efficient, robust, and scalable loading of EVs with fully stabilized hsiRNA conjugated with a cholesterol moiety without altering vesicle size distribution or integrity and promoting gene silencing in vivo [15]. Subsequently, exploiting the natural properties of EVs to functionally transport small RNAs [16–18] might offer an alternative solution for improving oligonucleotide in vivo distribution and cellular uptake [15, 19–26].

2 Materials

2.1 EVs Production and Purification

1. Tissue culture treated multilayer flask (e.g., T500 cm³ triple flask).
2. Phosphate-buffered saline (PBS).
3. Protease inhibitor cocktail stock solution (Sigma).
4. 70% Ethanol.
5. 50 ml conical centrifuge tubes.
6. Ultracentrifuge 70 ml polycarbonate bottles.
7. Fixed-angle Ti45 ultracentrifuge rotor (Beckman Coulter).
8. 1.5 ml microcentrifuge tubes.
9. 1.5 ml microcentrifuge adapters.
10. Fixed-angle TLA-110 rotor (Beckman Coulter).
11. Refrigerated centrifuge.
12. Refrigerated ultracentrifuge.

13. Refrigerated tabletop ultracentrifuge.

14. 0.22-μm filter-sterilization system.

15. 50 ml serological pipettes and pipetter.

16. Tips and micropipette.

17. Tissue culture hood connected to vacuum and tissue culture incubator.

18. −80 °C freezer.

19. Hamilton syringe.

20. HPLC system (e.g., Agilent 1100 HPLC).

2.2 EVs Loading and Characterization

1. Cy3-labeled or biotinylated cholesterol-conjugated hsiRNAs. Oligonucleotides are produced in-house. It is essential that compounds are significantly chemically stabilized with 2′-O-methyl and 2′-fluoro modifications in combination with a hydrophobic conjugate [15]. Sequences and chemical modification patterns of hsiRNAs used to develop this method are described in Table 1.

2. Cy3-OO-PNA stands fully complementary to the hsiRNAs guide strand (20 nucleotides long) (*PNA Bio*) (sequence and chemical modification pattern described in Table 1).

3. Purified EVs in PBS.

4. 1.5 ml microcentrifuge tubes.

5. 1.5 ml microcentrifuge adapters (Beckman Coulter).

6. Fixed-angle TLA-110 rotor (Beckman Coulter).

7. Orbital thermo-shaker for 1.5 ml microtube (e.g., PHMT Grant-Bio).

8. UV-transparent, flat-bottom 96-well plate.

9. Plate reader spectrophotometer (e.g., Infinite Pro1000, *Tecan*).

10. EVs size distribution and concentration reader (e.g., NanoSight NS300, *Malvern*).

11. 1 ml syringe.

12. Dip Cell kit (*Malvern, UK;* #ZEN1002).

13. Zetasizer Nano NS (*Malvern, UK*).

14. Anion exchange column (e.g., *Dionex* DNAPac PA100).

15. HPLC system with fluorescent detector, possibly autosampler.

16. ThermoCycler or heat block.

17. RIPA buffer (*Pierce* 899,000, *Thermo Fisher Scientific*) with 2 mg/ml proteinase K.

18. Electron microscopy grids and clean forceps to manipulate the grid.

19. Parafilm.

Table 1
Table describing hydrophobically modified hsiRNA target, sequences and modifications, and PNA strand

Target	Compounds				Conjugate
	Name	Type	Strand	Sequence 5′–3′	
Non-targeting control	hsiRNA[NTC]	hsiRNA	S	mA.mC.A.A.A.mU.A.mC.G.A.mU#mU#mA	Cholesterol
			AS	PmU.A.A.fU.fC.G.fU.A.fU.fU.G.mU#mC#A#A#mU#mC#A	
Huntingtin	hsiRNA[HTT]	hsiRNA	S	mC.mA.G.mU.A.A.A.mG.A.G.A.mU.mU#mA#mA	Cholesterol
			AS	PmU.fU.A.A.fU.fC.fU.fC.fU.fU.A.fC.fU#G#A#fU#A#fU#A	
Antisense hsiRNA[HTT]	PNA[HTT]	PNA	S	Cy3-OO-*T*A*T*A*T*C*A*G*T*A*A*A*T*A*G*A*T*T*A*A	None

S sense, *AS* antisense
m = 2′-*O*-methyl; f = 2′-fluoro; # = phosphorothioate; P = Phosphate; * = peptidyl interaction (*see* **Note 5**)

20. Whatman no. 1 filter paper.

21. EM grid storage boxes.

22. Transmission electron microscope (TEM).

2.3 Reagents and Solutions

1. Use ultrapure Milli-Q-purified water or equivalent in all recipes and protocol steps.

2. Culture medium for commonly used adherent cell lines such as U87 cells: Supplement 450 ml DMEM high glucose with 50 ml 100% FBS and 5 ml 100× penicillin-streptomycin.

3. 1 M sucrose: Dissolve 34.23 g of sucrose in 100 ml of distilled H_2O. Filter sterilize with 0.22-μm syringe filter and store at 4 °C.

4. 1 M Tris–HCl pH 8.5: Dissolve 121 g of Tris Base (TRIZMA) in 700 ml of distilled H_2O. Adjust the pH to 8.5 with HCl. Fill up to volume 1 L with distilled H_2O. Sterilize by autoclaving and store at room temperature.

5. HPLC buffer A: Dilute 50% acetonitrile, 25 mM Tris–HCl (pH 8.5), and 1 mM EDTA in water.

6. HPLC buffer B: Dilute 800 mM $NaClO_4$ in buffer A.

7. 0.5 M EDTA: Add 186.1 g of disodium EDTA (Na_2EDTA) in 800 ml of distilled H_2O. Adjust the pH to 8 with NaOH (~50 ml of NaOH). Bring the volume to 1 L with distilled H_2O. Mix on a magnetic stirrer. Sterilize by autoclaving and store at room temperature.

8. 3 M KCl: Dissolve 22.368 g of KCl in 100 ml of distilled H_2O and mix thoroughly.

9. 10% SDS: Dissolve 10 g of SDS in 80 ml of distilled H_2O. Adjust the volume to 100 ml with distilled water.

10. 0.1 M sodium phosphate buffer: Dilute 3.1 g of $NaH_2PO_4 \cdot H_2O$ and 10.9 g of Na_2HPO_4 (anhydrous) to distilled H_2O to make a volume of 1 L. This buffer can be stored for up to 1 month at 4 °C.

11. Glutaraldehyde, 1% (v/v): Dilute EM-grade glutaraldehyde fixatives (commercially available as 8%, 25%, or 70% aqueous solutions; Sigma) in 0.1 M sodium phosphate buffer, pH 7.4, to the appropriate dilution. Store up to 6 months at −20 °C or up to 1 week at 4 °C after thawing. The buffers used to prepare fixatives need to have a good buffering capacity to maintain a pH of about 7.4 during fixation.

12. Methyl cellulose, 2% (w/v): Heat 196 ml of distilled water to 90 °C and add 4 g methyl cellulose (Sigma) with stirring. Rapidly cool on ice with stirring, until the solution has reached 10 °C. Continue slow stirring overnight at 4 °C. Stop stirring and allow the solution "ripen" for 3 days at 4 °C. Bring to a final volume of 200 ml with water. Centrifuge using polycarbonate

centrifuge bottles with cap assemblies 95 min at 100,000 × *g*, 4 °C. Collect the supernatant and store up to 3 months at 4 °C.

13. Paraformaldehyde (PFA), 2% and 4% (w/v): Dissolve 4 g of PFA powder in 90 ml of 0.1 M sodium phosphate buffer and heat to 65 °C while stirring. If needed, add drops of 1 N NaOH until the solution becomes clear. Bring to 100 ml with 0.1 M sodium phosphate buffer. Cool and filter. Aliquot and store at −20 °C. Use thawed aliquots immediately and do not refreeze.

14. To make 2% glutaraldehyde, dilute 4% glutaraldehyde with 0.1 M sodium phosphate buffer.

15. Uranyl acetate (4% w/v), pH 4: Weigh 2 g of uranyl acetate and dissolve in 50 ml distilled water. Store up to 4 months at 4 °C protected from light. Just before use, filter the amount needed of uranyl solution with a 0.22-μm syringe filter. CAUTION: Consult with the institutional Radiation Safety Office for guidelines concerning proper handling and disposal of radioactive material. The uranyl acetate crystals are difficult to dissolve and it may be necessary to use a rotating wheel for mixing.

16. Uranyl oxalate, pH 7: Mix 4% uranyl acetate, pH 4 with 0.15 M oxalic acid (0.945 g in 50 ml distilled water), in a 1:1 ratio. Adjust the pH to 7 by adding 25% (w/v) NH_4OH in drops to prevent formation of insoluble precipitates. Store in the dark up to 1 month at 4 °C.

17. Methyl cellulose-UA, pH 4: nine parts 2% methyl cellulose and one part 4% uranyl acetate mixed just before use.

3   Methods

3.1   EVs Production and Purification

For in cellulo and in vivo efficacy experiments, sterile centrifuge and ultracentrifuge bottles and tubes are used. For EVs' production from cell culture and EVs' purification for biochemical analyses, such as immunoblot or proteomics, very clean bottles are required.

All manipulations with the open bottles must be performed in a tissue culture hood. To sterilize ultracentrifuge bottles, wash the bottles and their lids with soap using a soft brush and rinse with filtered water (multiple times). In a tissue culture hood, briefly soak the cleaned bottles and their lids in 70% ethanol and let dry on a paper towel, soaked with 70% ethanol. Perform a final sterilization in the tissue culture hood using the UV.

For all high-speed centrifugations, all 70 ml bottles should be full to the bottle shoulder (~65 ml). If one of the bottles is not filled to the bottle shoulder, complete the volume with PBS.

To indicate where to look for the pellet at the end of the ultra-centrifugation using 70 ml polycarbonate bottles, mark a side of each bottle with a marker, and orient the bottles in the centrifuge with mark facing up.

3.1.1   Preparing EV-Free Medium and Cell Culture

To collect large quantities of EVs (e.g., for in vivo experiments), we purify EVs from EV-containing conditioned medium from adherent cells in culture. The yield of purified EVs increases with the increase of starting volume of conditioned medium. Thus, to scale up the cells number and produce at least 360 ml of conditioned medium, we use a minimum of six T500 cm^3 triple flasks. However, EVs are present in the serum generally used to supplement cell culture medium. Thus, to avoid contamination by these EVs, the culture medium used to grow cells from which the EVs will be purified must be depleted of the contaminating serum-EVs.

1. For each cell line, prepare the recommended medium supplemented with 40% (v/v) FBS. *Depleting medium supplemented with 40% FBS allows preparation of a large volume of EV-free culture medium in a single round of centrifugation.*

2. Transfer the medium in 70 ml polycarbonate bottles and centrifuge overnight at 100,000 × *g*, 4 °C using a Type 45 Ti rotor (*see* **Note 1**).

3. Transfer the contents of each bottle into a vacuum-connected 0.22-μm filter-sterile bottle unit using a 50 ml serological pipette to filter sterilize the supernatant (i.e., depleted medium). At the bottom of the bottle, leave 2–3 ml of medium containing higher concentration of brown sediment that pelleted during the ultracentrifugation. The pellet is brown and very sticky and should not be detached from the edge of the bottle.

4. Prior to cell culture, dilute the EVs-depleted medium with additional medium to reach the final FBS concentration (usually 10% FBS) required for the cell culture and supplement with all the nutrients and antibiotics necessary.

5. Store the sterilized EVs-depleted medium, diluted or not, up to 4 weeks at 4 °C.

6. Grow adherent cells of interest in 60 ml of recommended medium until they reach 70–80% confluency in as much T500 cm^3 triple flask as necessary.

7. Remove the culture medium, and replace it with a similar volume of recommended EV-depleted medium.

8. Culture the cells for 48 h at 37 °C, 5% CO_2 and 100% humidity.

9. If the cells are not at 100% confluency, replace the collected medium with fresh EV-depleted medium, culture for 48 h, and proceed to EVs purification as followed.

3.1.2 Purification of EVs

EVs were purified from conditioned medium by a method adapted from Thery et al. and combining sequential centrifugation and filtration steps (*see* **Note 2**) [27]. All EVs quality controls were performed following recommended experimental requirement [27, 28].

1. Harvest the conditioned culture medium containing EVs in 50 ml centrifuge conical tubes and centrifuge at 300 × *g* for 10 min at room temperature to eliminate cells.

2. Transfer the supernatant into new 50 ml centrifuge conical tubes using 50 ml serological pipette. Leave 2–3 ml of medium in the bottom of the tube to avoid disturbing the pellet. Discard the pellet.

3. Centrifuge the supernatant at 10,000 × *g*, 4 °C for 30 min to eliminate large cell debris.

The resulting pellet, containing microvesicles, is white, very sticky and can be saved for additional experiments involving microvesicles.

4. Pour and filter sterilize the supernatant through a vacuum-connected 0.22-μm filter on top of a sterile bottle to eliminate large cell debris and membranes.

5. Transfer the filtered medium in 70 ml polycarbonate bottles and ultracentrifuge for at least 70 min at 100,000 × *g*, 4 °C using a Type 45 Ti rotor.

6. Aspirate the supernatant completely from all bottles using a vacuum-connected Pasteur pipette.

Remaining medium will fall down the edge of the bottle and form a final drop of supernatant that has to be aspirated by vacuum-connected Pasteur pipette.

7. To concentrate the EVs, suspend all the pellets in the same 1 ml PBS using a micropipette. Scratch the edge of the bottle in and around the pellet with the tip to recover a maximum of EVs.

8. Transfer the suspended pellet into 1.5 ml microcentrifuge tube.

9. Place the tubes in the tube holder and then the tube holder in the rotor with the tube-cap orientated to find the pellet.

10. Centrifuge for at least 70 min at 100,000 × *g*, 4 °C in a tabletop ultracentrifuge using a TLA-110 rotor.

11. Suspend the pellet in 100 μl PBS for further experiments (*see* **Note 3**). Save an aliquot of EVs for measurement of EVs size and concentration by NTA (*see* **Note 4**).

For storage at −80 °C for up to 6 months, suspend the pellet in 100 μl PBS supplemented with 1 μl protease inhibitor cocktail 100× and 10 μl of 1 M sucrose (final concentration 100 mM). Avoid repeated freezing and thawing.

For proteomic or lipidomic analysis, store the pellet as is at −80°C.

3.2 EVs Loading with hsiRNAs and Characterization of hsiRNA-Loaded EVs

3.2.1 Loading of EVs with Hydrophobic siRNAs (hsiRNAs)

The loading of EVs with hsiRNA is performed as shown in Fig. 1 (*see* **Notes 5** and **6**).

1. Into a 1.5 ml microcentrifuge tube, mix required concentration of hsiRNAs with EVs suspended in PBS by pipetting up and down with micropipette.

2. Incubate the mix for at least 60 min at 37 °C and shaking at 500 rpm. If the oligonucleotide is fluorescently labeled, protect the tube from light.

3. Place the tubes in the tube holder and in the rotor with the tube-cap orientated to find the pellet.

4. Centrifuge for at least 70 min at $100,000 \times g$, 4 °C in a tabletop ultracentrifuge using a TLA-110 rotor. hsiRNA-loaded EVs form a pellet while unloaded hsiRNAs remain in the supernatant.

5. Remove and save the supernatant into a 1.5 ml centrifugation for further measurement. The unloaded hsiRNAs remain in the supernatant, and quantification of hsiRNA remaining in supernatant can be used to estimate the efficiency of loading (for quantification of hsiRNA concentration, *see* Subheadings 3.2.2 and 3.2.3).

6. Suspend the pellet in required volume of medium for in cellulo experiments or aCSF for in vivo brain injection. The pellet can be suspended in PBS depending on the following experiments. hsiRNA-loaded EVs are immediately used for further experiment without being stored (*see* **Note 7**).

7. Save an aliquot of hsiRNA-loaded EVs for measurement of hsiRNA and EVs concentration.

3.2.2 Determination of hsiRNA Concentration by Direct Quantification of Fluorescently Labeled hsiRNAs

The loading efficiency of hsiRNAs in EVs is estimated by two methods (Fig. 1) (*see* **Note 8**). First, by directly measuring the Cy3 fluorescence in the hsiRNA-EVs pellet. Second, by calculating the difference between the total amount of Cy3-hsiRNA originally added to the sample and the amount of Cy3-hsiRNA remaining in the supernatant after EVs incubation and ultracentrifugation. To determine accurate concentration of hsiRNAs, prepare negative controls and a hsiRNAs calibration curve into the well of a UV-transparent, flat-bottom 96-well plate.

1. Dispense 50 μl of PBS in the first well as a negative control (blank).

2. In the following well, prepare a Cy3 fluorescent positive control stock solution by diluting Cy3-labeled hsiRNAs in 100 μl PBS.

3. Dispense 50 μl of PBS into three following wells. To make a series dilution, transfer 50 μl of the stock solution into the next well containing 50 μl of PBS and mix.

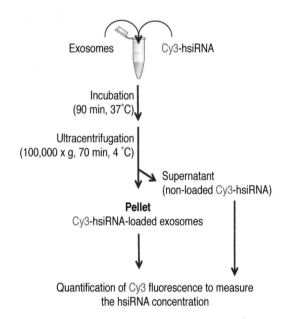

Fig. 1 Flowchart of exosome loading procedure: co-incubation of Cy3-hsiRNA and exosomes results in Cy3-hsiRNA-loaded exosomes that pellet by ultracentrifugation

4. Using a fresh pipet tip, transfer 50 μl into the next well and proceed until the last well of the calibration curve.

5. Transfer 50 μl of supernatant (containing unloaded hsiRNA) and pellet (containing hsiRNA-EVs) of each sample into the plate.

6. Read the Cy3 fluorescence using a spectrophotometer plate-reader at 547 nm excitation and 570 nm emission wavelengths.

7. Using the calibration curve, estimate directly the Cy3 fluorescence in the pellet samples.

8. In addition, using the calibration curve, estimate the Cy3 fluorescence remaining in the supernatant. To estimate the concentration of hsiRNAs in the pellet by a second method, calculate the difference between the total amount Cy3-hsiRNAs originally added to the sample and the amount of Cy3 fluorescence remaining in the supernatant (*see* **Note 9**).

3.2.3 Determination of hsiRNA Concentration by Peptide-Nucleic Acid Hybridization Assay

To confirm the quantification of hsiRNAs obtained by measuring the Cy3 fluorescence of pellet using a spectrophotometer, we determine the hsiRNAs guide strand concentration in samples using a peptide-nucleic acid (PNA) hybridization assay (developed by *Axolabs GmbH, Kulmbach, Germany*) [29]. PNAs are single strand analogues of DNA in which the sugar-phosphate backbone is replaced with a polyamide backbone (Table 1). PNAs therefore carry no charge and bind to their complementary strand with very high affinity, invading double-stranded DNA and RNA structures.

1. Dilute hsiRNA-loaded EVs sample pellet in 100 µl of radioimmunoprecipitation assay (RIPA) buffer containing 2 mg/ml proteinase K and sonicate for 15 min for vesicle lysis.

2. Centrifuge sample for 15 min at $16,000 \times g$ in tabletop centrifuge to pellet out non-soluable membrane material and transfer supernatant containing hsiRNA into a fresh microcentrifuge tube.

3. To prepare a calibration curve, add a known amount of hsiRNA duplex into lysed EVs sample.

4. Add 20 µl of 3 M KCl and centrifuge at $5,000 \times g$, 4 °C to precipitate the SDS (from RIPA buffer).

5. Transfer the cleared supernatant containing the hsiRNAs guide strands in a new 1.5 ml microcentrifuge tube.

6. Dilute supernatant to reach an estimated concentration below 5 pmol hsiRNA/100 µl sample. Then add 5 pmol of Cy3-labeled PNA strands fully complementary to guide strand of hsiRNA.

1. Anneal PNA to hsiRNA guide strand: incubate at 95 °C for 15 min followed by incubation at 50 °C for 15 min and cool to room temperature.

2. Transfer all the samples in a 96-well plate or vials compatible with your HPLC system.

3. Inject the samples containing hsiRNA guide strand-PNA hybrids into HPLC anion exchange column (Dionex DNAPac PA100) using an autosampler or manually using a Hamilton syringe. The mobile phase for HPLC is as follows: buffer A, 50% acetonitrile, 25 mM Tris–HCl (pH 8.5), and 1 mM EDTA in water; buffer B, 800 mM $NaClO_4$ in buffer A. Optimize speed of gradient between 10% buffer B and 100% buffer B to your HPLC system and anion exchange column.

An example:

0 min	90% A, 10% B	
2 min	90% A, 10% B	Equilibration, free PNA should come around 2 min (void volume)
10 min	50% A, 50% B	Elution, PNA-hsiRNA hybrid should come around 40% B, 7.5–8.5 min
10.5 min	100% B	
12.5 min	100%B	Wash
13 min	90% A, 10% B	
15 min	90% A, 10% B	Regeneration

4. Read the Cy3 fluorescence (excitation 550 nm, emission 570 nm) and integrate peak corresponding to PNA-hsiRNA guide strand hybrid.

5. Calculate the hsiRNA guide strand concentration using the calibration curve.

3.2.4 Characterization of EVs Size Distribution and Concentration

For each sample, the concentration and size of particles is determined by recording and analyzing the Brownian motion of particles using a NanoSight NS300 system and Nanoparticles Tracking Analysis software (*Malvern, UK*).

1. Dilute 1–5 μl of sample in 1 ml PBS (dilution ratio 1:200 to 1:1000) at room temperature in a 1.5 ml microtube and mix gently using 1 ml micropipette.

2. Inject the diluted sample in the NanoSight NS300 system using a clean 1 ml syringe.

3. Adjust camera shutter and gain manually.

4. Monitor the sample in duplicate for 30–60 s.

5. Analyze the recorded videos using the Nanoparticle Tracking Analysis (NTA) software to determine the particle size and concentration.

6. Determine the number of hsiRNAs loaded *per* EV by dividing the total amount of hsiRNAs in the sample by the number of EVs detected by NTA, assuming normal distribution.

3.2.5 Characterization of EVs Surface Charge

The hsiRNA-loaded EVs surface charges are determined by Laser Doppler Micro-electrophoresis (DLM).

1. Dilute 1 to 5 μl of sample in 1 ml distilled H_2O (dilution ratio 1:200 to 1:1000) at room temperature in a 1.5 ml microtube and mix gently using 1 ml micropipette.

The particles' charge determined by applying an electric field to the solution of molecules, which then move with a velocity related to their surface charges. We noticed that diluting the sample in PBS provoked the burn of the solution inducing false measurements.

1. Transfer the diluted sample in a universal glass micro-electrophoresis cuvette.

2. Monitor the sample charges in duplicate.

3. The instrument gives absolute values of particles charges.

We observed that hsiRNA-loaded EVs have lower negative charges than non-loaded EVs.

3.2.6 Analysis of hsiRNA-Loaded EVs Integrity by Electron Microscopy

To detect hsiRNAs bound to EVs by electron microscopy, we use biotinylated hsiRNA. Samples and grids for electron microscopy were prepared at room temperature unless otherwise specified.

1. Add an equal volume of 4% paraformaldehyde to the hsiRNA-loaded EV sample and incubate for 2 h.

2. Drop 3 μl of fixed hsiRNA-loaded EV aliquots onto EM grids.

3. Incubate for 20 min in a dry environment to let the membrane adsorb.

4. To wash the grid, drop 100 μl of PBS on a sheet of parafilm and transfer the grids to the drop of PBS. The membrane should be side down.

5. Subsequent steps are performed similarly, transferring the grid from drop to drop of reagents on a sheet of parafilm.

6. Transfer the grid to a 100 μl drop of 50 mM glycine/PBS and incubate for 5 min.

7. Transfer the grid to a 100 μl drop of 5% BSA/PBS for 10 min to block the sample.

8. The addition of 0.1% saponin to the reagent will permeabilize the EVs to enable the detection of any intraluminal hsiRNA molecule.

9. Wash the grid twice in PBS.

10. Incubate the grid with 50 μl drop of 6- or 10-nm streptavidin immune-gold particles diluted 1:10 to 1:20 in 0.5% BSA/PBS for 1 h in presence or absence of 0.1% saponin.

11. Wash the grid three times in PBS.

12. Incubate the grid in 1% glutaraldehyde for 5 min.

13. Wash the grid eight times in water of 2 min each wash.

14. Transfer the grid in uranyl oxalate pH 7 for 5 min to contrast the sample.

15. Contrast and embed the samples in a 9:1 solution of respectively 1% methyl cellulose and 4% uranyl acetate for 10 min on ice.

16. Remove the excess liquid with a Whatman no. 1 filter paper and let the grids air-dried for 5–10 min.

17. Observe the grid in a transmission electron microscope at 60–80 kV.

18. Store the grid in an appropriate environment.

4   Notes

1. After ultracentrifugation of EV-depleted medium, EVs or hsiRNA-loaded EVs, it is important to remove the supernatant quickly to avoid the pellet to dissolve back in the supernatant.

2. We find that it is best to prepare fresh EVs whenever possible for each functional in vitro and in vivo assay.

3. Purified EVs are kept at 4 °C for a maximum of 48 h prior any functional assay.

4. In addition to NTA, the measurement of protein concentration of purified EVs represents a reproducible approach to quantify EVs.

5. Particular attention should be given to the hsiRNAs modification pattern. Functionally efficient hsiRNA-loaded EVs require extensive chemical stabilization of hsiRNAs. Riboses chemically modified with 2′-O-methyl and 2′-fluoro modifications result in significant hsiRNA-resistance to nuclease degradation and provide high stability in vitro and in vivo. Partially modified hsiRNAs may undergo degradation *via* nucleases, originating potentially from the EVs sample purified from conditioned cell culture medium, and thus will affect hsiRNAs and hsiRNA-loaded EVs functional efficacy.

6. The co-incubation of cholesterol-conjugated hsiRNAs with EVs provides a robust, efficient, and highly reproducible method for loading EVs with chemically synthesized oligonucleotides. We observed that the cholesterol is essential for loading as non-cholesterol-conjugated hsiRNAs did not associate with exosomes [15]. We used the same procedure to load EVs with siRNAs conjugated to various hydrophobic moiety (e.g., DHA). We observed that the more hydrophobic is the conjugate, the more efficient is the loading (data not published).

7. Chemical modifications of hsiRNAs provide resistance against nucleases, independent of localization of the EV-loaded hsiRNA (i.e. inside the vesicle or externally bound). But, at this point, we cannot define which of the EVs-associated oligonucleotides (surface bound or internalized) are functionally active. Further studies are essential to determine the optimal loading, long-term stability, and in vivo behavior of the hsiRNA-loaded exosomes.

8. We noticed that EVs purified from different cell sources (e.g., glioblastoma-, mesenchymal stem cell- or umbilical-derived EVs) show similar ability to be loaded with hsiRNAs.

9. The loading of EVs with hsiRNA is saturable with maximum of ~ 3000–5000 hsiRNA loaded *per* individual vesicle. However, incubation of EVs with higher concentration of hsiRNAs slightly increases the number of hsiRNAs *per* EV. With increase in the hsiRNA/vesicle loading ratio, there is a slight increase in surface negative charge indicative of the hsiRNAs association with the vesicle membrane. Thus, it is possible that too much loading might interfere with native EVs cellular uptake mechanism.

Acknowledgments

We thank the members of the Khvorova and Aronin Laboratories, NIH Extracellular RNA Consortium and CHDI Foundation Inc. for helpful discussions. This work is supported in part NIH UH2-UH3 grant TR 000888 05 to N.A. and A.K., NIH grants RO1GM10880304, RO1NS10402201, and S10 OD020012 to A.K. and CHDI Foundation (Research Agreement A-6119, JSC A6367) to N.A. Marie-Cecile Didiot was supported by Huntington's Disease Society of America Postdoctoral Fellowship. The authors declare no conflict of interest.

References

1. Khvorova A, Watts JK (2017) The chemical evolution of oligonucleotide therapies of clinical utility. Nat Biotechnol 35(3):238–248. https://doi.org/10.1038/nbt.3765

2. Byrne M, Tzekov R, Wang Y, Rodgers A, Cardia J, Ford G, Holton K, Pandarinathan L, Lapierre J, Stanney W, Bulock K, Shaw S, Libertine L, Fettes K, Khvorova A, Kaushal S, Pavco P (2013) Novel hydrophobically modified asymmetric RNAi compounds (sd-rxRNA) demonstrate robust efficacy in the eye. J Ocul Pharmacol Ther 29(10):855–864. https://doi.org/10.1089/jop.2013.0148

3. Geary RS, Norris D, Yu R, Bennett CF (2015) Pharmacokinetics, biodistribution and cell uptake of antisense oligonucleotides. Adv Drug Deliv Rev 87:46–51. https://doi.org/10.1016/j.addr.2015.01.008

4. Alterman JF, Hall LM, Coles AH, Hassler MR, Didiot MC, Chase K, Abraham J, Sottosanti E, Johnson E, Sapp E, Osborn MF, Difiglia M, Aronin N, Khvorova A (2015) Hydrophobically modified siRNAs silence huntingtin mRNA in primary neurons and mouse brain. Mol Ther Nucleic Acids 4:e266. https://doi.org/10.1038/mtna.2015.38

5. Ly S, Navaroli D, Didiot M, Cardia J, Pandarinathan L, Alterman J, Fogarty K, Standley C, Lifshitz L, Bellve K, Prot M, Echeverria D, Corvera S, Khvorova A (2016) Visualization of self-delivering hydrophobically modified siRNA cellular internalization. Nucleic Acids Res. https://doi.org/10.1093/nar/gkw1005

6. Distler JH, Huber LC, Hueber AJ, Reich CF 3rd, Gay S, Distler O, Pisetsky DS (2005) The release of microparticles by apoptotic cells and their effects on macrophages. Apoptosis 10(4):731–741. https://doi.org/10.1007/s10495-005-2941-5

7. Muralidharan-Chari V, Clancy JW, Sedgwick A, D'Souza-Schorey C (2010) Microvesicles: mediators of extracellular communication during cancer progression. J Cell Sci 123(Pt 10):1603–1611. https://doi.org/10.1242/jcs.064386

8. Tetta C, Ghigo E, Silengo L, Deregibus MC, Camussi G (2013) Extracellular vesicles as an emerging mechanism of cell-to-cell communication. Endocrine 44(1):11–19. https://doi.org/10.1007/s12020-012-9839-0

9. Alvarez-Erviti L, Seow Y, Yin H, Betts C, Lakhal S, Wood MJ (2011) Delivery of siRNA to the mouse brain by systemic injection of targeted exosomes. Nat Biotechnol 29(4):341–345. https://doi.org/10.1038/nbt.1807

10. Cooper JM, Wiklander PB, Nordin JZ, Al-Shawi R, Wood MJ, Vithlani M, Schapira AH, Simons JP, El-Andaloussi S, Alvarez-Erviti L (2014) Systemic exosomal siRNA delivery reduced alpha-synuclein aggregates in brains of transgenic mice. Mov Disord 29(12):1476–1485. https://doi.org/10.1002/mds.25978

11. Ohno S, Takanashi M, Sudo K, Ueda S, Ishikawa A, Matsuyama N, Fujita K, Mizutani T, Ohgi T, Ochiya T, Gotoh N, Kuroda M (2013) Systemically injected exosomes targeted to EGFR deliver antitumor microRNA to breast cancer cells. Mol Ther 21(1):185–191. https://doi.org/10.1038/mt.2012.180

12. Mizrak A, Bolukbasi MF, Ozdener GB, Brenner GJ, Madlener S, Erkan EP, Strobel T, Breakefield XO, Saydam O (2013) Genetically engineered microvesicles carrying suicide mRNA/protein inhibit schwannoma tumor growth. Mol Ther 21(1):101–108. https://doi.org/10.1038/mt.2012.161

13. Kosaka N, Iguchi H, Yoshioka Y, Hagiwara K, Takeshita F, Ochiya T (2012) Competitive interactions of cancer cells and normal cells via

secretory microRNAs. J Biol Chem 287(2):1397–1405. https://doi.org/10.1074/jbc.M111.288662

14. Kooijmans SA, Stremersch S, Braeckmans K, de Smedt SC, Hendrix A, Wood MJ, Schiffelers RM, Raemdonck K, Vader P (2013) Electroporation-induced siRNA precipitation obscures the efficiency of siRNA loading into extracellular vesicles. J Control Release 172(1):229–238. https://doi.org/10.1016/j.jconrel.2013.08.014

15. Didiot MC, Hall LM, Coles AH, Haraszti RA, Godinho BM, Chase K, Sapp E, Ly S, Alterman JF, Hassler MR, Echeverria D, Raj L, Morrissey DV, DiFiglia M, Aronin N, Khvorova A (2016) Exosome-mediated delivery of hydrophobically modified siRNA for huntingtin mRNA silencing. Mol Ther. https://doi.org/10.1038/mt.2016.126

16. Wang K, Zhang S, Weber J, Baxter D, Galas DJ (2010) Export of microRNAs and microRNA-protective protein by mammalian cells. Nucleic Acids Res 38(20):7248–7259. https://doi.org/10.1093/nar/gkq601

17. Pegtel DM, Cosmopoulos K, Thorley-Lawson DA, van Eijndhoven MA, Hopmans ES, Lindenberg JL, de Gruijl TD, Wurdinger T, Middeldorp JM (2010) Functional delivery of viral miRNAs via exosomes. Proc Natl Acad Sci U S A 107(14):6328–6333. https://doi.org/10.1073/pnas.0914843107

18. Valadi H, Ekstrom K, Bossios A, Sjostrand M, Lee JJ, Lotvall JO (2007) Exosome-mediated transfer of mRNAs and microRNAs is a novel mechanism of genetic exchange between cells. Nat Cell Biol 9(6):654–659. https://doi.org/10.1038/ncb1596

19. El Andaloussi S, Lakhal S, Mager I, Wood MJ (2013) Exosomes for targeted siRNA delivery across biological barriers. Adv Drug Deliv Rev 65(3):391–397. https://doi.org/10.1016/j.addr.2012.08.008

20. Kooijmans SA, Vader P, van Dommelen SM, van Solinge WW, Schiffelers RM (2012) Exosome mimetics: a novel class of drug delivery systems. Int J Nanomedicine 7:1525–1541. https://doi.org/10.2147/IJN.S29661

21. Pan Q, Ramakrishnaiah V, Henry S, Fouraschen S, de Ruiter PE, Kwekkeboom J, Tilanus HW, Janssen HL, van der Laan LJ (2012) Hepatic cell-to-cell transmission of small silencing RNA can extend the therapeutic reach of RNA interference (RNAi). Gut 61(9):1330–1339. https://doi.org/10.1136/gutjnl-2011-300449

22. Lasser C (2012) Exosomal RNA as biomarkers and the therapeutic potential of exosome vectors. Expert Opin Biol Ther 12(Suppl 1):S189–S197. https://doi.org/10.1517/14712598.2012.680018

23. Lee Y, El Andaloussi S, Wood MJ (2012) Exosomes and microvesicles: extracellular vesicles for genetic information transfer and gene therapy. Hum Mol Genet 21(R1):R125–R134. https://doi.org/10.1093/hmg/dds317

24. Marcus ME, Leonard JN (2013) FedExosomes: engineering therapeutic biological nanoparticles that truly deliver. Pharmaceuticals (Basel) 6(5):659–680. https://doi.org/10.3390/ph6050659

25. Nazarenko I, Rupp AK, Altevogt P (2013) Exosomes as a potential tool for a specific delivery of functional molecules. Methods Mol Biol 1049:495–511. https://doi.org/10.1007/978-1-62703-547-7_37

26. Zomer A, Vendrig T, Hopmans ES, van Eijndhoven M, Middeldorp JM, Pegtel DM (2010) Exosomes: fit to deliver small RNA. Commun Integr Biol 3(5):447–450. https://doi.org/10.4161/cib.3.5.12339

27. Thery C, Amigorena S, Raposo G, Clayton A (2006) Isolation and characterization of exosomes from cell culture supernatants and biological fluids. Curr Protoc Cell Biol. Chapter 3:Unit 3.22. https://doi.org/10.1002/0471143030.cb0322s30

28. Lotvall J, Hill AF, Hochberg F, Buzas EI, Di Vizio D, Gardiner C, Gho YS, Kurochkin IV, Mathivanan S, Quesenberry P, Sahoo S, Tahara H, Wauben MH, Witwer KW, Thery C (2014) Minimal experimental requirements for definition of extracellular vesicles and their functions: a position statement from the International Society for Extracellular Vesicles. J Extracell Vesicles 3:26913. https://doi.org/10.3402/jev.v3.26913

29. Roehl I, Schuster M, Seiffert S (2011) Oligonucleotide detection method. US Patent Application US20110201006A1

INDEX

Tushar Patel (ed.), *Extracellular RNA: Methods and Protocols*, Methods in Molecular Biology, vol. 1740,
https://doi.org/10.1007/978-1-4939-7652-2, © Springer Science+Business Media, LLC 2018

215

Printed in the United States
By Bookmasters